2020 Keto Foodi Pressure

Delicious & Easy to Prepare Low Carb Foodi Recipes and Effective Weight Loss Tips on the Ketogenic Diet to Keep you Fit in 2020

By Mariana Cleff

Copyright © 2019 by Mariana Cleff

All rights reserved worldwide. You may not reproduce or transmitted any part of the book, in any form or by any means, electronic or mechanical, including photocopying, recording or by any information storage and retrieval system, without written permission from the publisher or author, except for the inclusion of brief quotations in a review.

Table of Contents

DISCLAIMER ....ERROR! BOOKMARK NOT DEFINED.

TABLE OF CONTENTS... 2

INTRODUCTION 12

CHAPTER ONE: INTRODUCTION TO NINJA FOODI 13

How Ninja Foodi Work 14

Rules for Using the Ninja Foodi 15

Function Buttons in Foodi Crisping Pressure................................... 16

What You Can Do with Ninja Foodi.. 19

How to Use the Foodi Crisping Pressure Cooker 20

Cleaning & Maintenance of Your Foodi Pressure cooker 21

Removing & Reinstalling the Silicone Ring...................................... 22

Useful Tips for Your Foodi Crisping Pressure cooker 22

Ninja Foodi Cook Settings 24

Foodi Air Crisp Conversion Chart 25

Foodi Pressure Cooker Chart 26

CHAPTER TWO: RECIPE CONVERSION TABLE 28

Ninja Foodi Cook Settings 28

Foodi Air Crisp Conversion Chart 29

Foodi Pressure Cooker Chart 30

CHAPTER THREE: INTRODUCTION TO KETO.. 32

What is the Ketogenic Diet? 32

How to Lose Weight with the Ketogenic Diet?...33

Keto Friendly Foods..35

Foods to Avoid on Keto Diet 37

FAQS About Keto Diet 39

CHAPTER FOUR: KETO NINJA FOODI BREAKFAST RECIPES 41

Tomato Cups 41

Savory Cheese and Ham Custard 43

Keto egg bites...45

Veggie Frittata..46

Pumpkin Spice Breakfast Cake 48

Zucchini Egg Cups 49

Parmesan Chicken Wings 50

Feta Frittata 52

Pancetta Hash with Baked Eggs 53

Avocado Bacon Bombs 54

Tortilla Ham Wraps 55

Raspberry Breakfast Cake..57

Cauliflower Hash browns 59

Egg Crumpet Sandwiches	60
Cheesy Chorizo Topping	62
Spinach Muffins	64
Bacon and Egg Bites	65
Mason Jar Omelet	66
Cinnamon Chia Pudding	67
Veggie Egg Casserole	68
Ham and Eggs Casserole	69
Fish with Sesame	70
Delightful Cheese Casserole	71
Bacon, Broccoli and Cheddar Frittata	73
Coconut Oatmeal	74
Spicy Bacon Bites	75
Almond Muffins	76
Artichoke Frittata	77
Stuffed Buns with Egg	79
Bacon, Avocado and Cheese	80
Cheesy Hash	81
Cheese Casserole	82
Western Omelet	83
Creamy Early Morning Asparagus Soup	84
Amazing Bacon and Veggie Delight	86

Quiche Lorainde 87

Bacon Jalapeno 88

Egg Caprese Breakfast Cups 89

CHAPTER FIVE: CHICKEN AND POULTRY RECIPES 90

Juicy Sesame Garlic Chicken Wings 90

Chicken Salad in Jar 92

Tomato Chicken Stew 94

Chicken Puttanesca 96

Spicy Chicken Strips 98

Fragrant Drumsticks 101

Chicken Soup 102

Dill Chicken Wings 103

Lemon and Butter Chicken Extravagant 104

Salsa Verde Chicken 105

Cheddar Chicken Fillets 106

Thai Chicken Fillet 108

BBQ Chicken Balls 109

Stuffed Chicken Caprese 110

Breast with Pomegranate Sauce 112

Spicy Hot Paprika Chicken 114

Oregano Chicken Wings 116

Chicken Bread 117

Crunchy Chicken Skin 119

Chicken Nuggets 120

Sour Cream Chicken Liver 121

Ham-Stuffed Generous Turkey Rolls 122

Shredded Chicken in Lettuce 123

Sensational Lime and Chicken Chili 124

Aromatic Whole Chicken 125

Funky-Garlic And turkey Breasts 127

Chicken Jerky 128

Sweet and Sour Chicken Wings 129

Steamed Chicken Cutlets 130

CHAPTER SIX: KETO NINJA FOODI APPETIZERS AND DESERTS 131

Glazed Walnuts 131

Blackberry Cake 132

Avocado Mousse 133

Cheesy Bombs 134

Cashew Cream 135

Broccoli Tots 136

Meatloaf 137

Garlic Tomato Slices 138

Coconut Pie 139

Wrapped Halloumi Cheese 140

Lava Cups	141
Peanut Butter Cookies	142
Spinach Dip	143
Cauliflower Fritters	144
Keto Brownie Batter	146
Breadsticks	147
Almond Bites	148
Ginger Cookies	149
Mini Cheese Cakes	150
Vanilla Crème Brulee	151
Delicious Lemon Mousse	152
Cinnamon Bun	153
Pumpkin Muffins	154
Chocolate Cakes	155
Keto Donuts	156
Keto Brownie	157
Pumpkin Pie	158
Hearty Carrot Pumpkin Pudding	159
Artichoke Dip	161
Loaded Nachos	162
Buffalo Cauliflower Bites	163
Jicama Fries	165

The Original Pot-De-Crème 166

CHAPTER SEVEN: KETO NINJA FOODI VEGAN AND VEGETARIAN 167

Cauliflower Puree with Scallions 167

Garlic and Dill Carrot Fiesta 169

Zucchini Gratin 170

Asian-Style Asparagus and Tofu Scramble 171

Zucchini Pizza 173

Steamed Kale 174

Quinoa with Veggies 175

Roasted Green Beans with Lime Juice 176

Hot and Spicy Black Beans 177

Astounding Caramelized Onions 179

Herb Carrots 180

Summertime Veggie Soup 181

Delicious Mushroom Stroganoff 183

Offbeat Cauliflower and Cheddar Soup 184

Medi-Cheese Spinach 185

Butternut Squash Soup 186

Zucchini Fries 188

Bacon and Cabbage 189

Spicy Green Beans 190

Kale Chips 191

CHAPTER EIGHT: KETO NINJA FOODI SEAFOOD RECIPES 192

Herby Cods 192

Salmon and Balsamic Shallots 193

Marjoram Salmon 194

Tender Octopus 195

Fish Curry 196

Calamari in Tomato Sauce 198

Tomato and Shrimp Medley 200

The Smoked White Fish 201

Seafood Paella 203

Lemony Tuna Bites 205

Cool Lemon and Dill Fish Packages 206

Fish Pie 207

Cumin Mackerel Fillets 209

Spicy Whitebait 210

Heart-Throb Buttery Scallops 212

Shrimp and Peas 213

Coconut Fish Curry 214

Monkfish Stew 216

Warm Cajun Bass Stew 218

Cilantro Cod 220

The Great Lobster Bisque 221

Sriracha Shrimp 223

Elegant Fish Curry 224

Almond Cod Fillets 225

Tuna and Shirataki Noodles Salad 226

Cod with Broccoli, Lemon and Dill Mismash 228

Cod and Celery Stew 229

Crunchy Cod 230

Butter Dredged "Rich" Lobster 231

Shrimp and Tomatoes 232

Spicy Flounder 233

Lemon Pepper Salmon 234

CHAPTER NINE: KETO NINJA FOODI PORK AND BEEF RECIPES 235

Beef Jerky 235

Baked Thyme Pork Stew 236

Pork and Adobo Sauce 237

Beef Stew 238

Beef Ragout 239

Pork Chops and Basil Pesto 241

Beef Stifado 242

Beef Ribs 244

Lamb and Butternut Squash 246

Beef and Brussels Sprouts 247

NY Strip Steak 248

Beef Brisket with Red Wine 249

Pork and Sweet Onion 250

Short Ribs and Veggies 251

Parmesan Beef Meatloaf 253

Pork and Red Cabbage 255

Cauliflower Corned Beef Harsh 256

Ropa Vieja 257

Lemon Pork Chops 258

Sliced Beef with Saffron 259

Pork with the Almonds and Sage 261

Pork Schnitzel 262

Crazy Greek Lamb Gyros 263

CONCLUSION 264

Mariana Cleff

Introduction

A ketogenic diet is a way of eating that is very low in carbohydrates. Reducing carbs changes the body's metabolism and is perfect for easy weight loss. The metabolic process burns fat when it doesn't have enough carbohydrates.

Being on the ketogenic diet isn't entirely comfortable in a society that is heavy-carb obsessed. Hence, relying on easy cooking processes, availability of ingredients, and the quickness to make tasty food are my ways of winning daily. I have found the Ninja Foodi to boost my satisfaction! It offers excellent results on time and quality as compared to the pressure cooker and air fryer combined. These are the kind of treats that make me spend!

Have you ever dreamed of a device that could replace four or even five kitchen machines? I am sure that you are most likely familiar with the lack of space to put all the appliances in the kitchen and make it comfortable for yourself. a pressure cooker is a unique miracle machine that has many talents. Imagine that now you don't need to buy a slow cooker, pressure cooker, rice cooker, steamer, yogurt machine, or any other useful pots - all these functions already exist in this multitalented device. A pressure cooker is easy to use and take care of. This is the perfect solution for big families, busy people, and those who are not ready to spend a huge amount of time near the stove and want to devote this time to themselves and their loved ones.

If you are new to the keto diet or been on it for a while, but feeling a bit overwhelmed by finding recipes and spending too much time cooking them, then this book is for you. Not because I'm the author, but because I spent months testing these recipes and trying them consistently with the Ninja Foodi to be sure they are perfect. And they rock!

This book is a guide to the Ketogenic diet for beginners and to using the Ninja Foodi cooking device. It contains about 1000 Ketogenic Recipes you can prepare on your Ninja Foodi (Breakfasts, Snacks, Appetizers, Desserts, Sea foods, Vegan and Vegetarian, Chicken and Poultry, Beef and pork Recipes)

Chapter One: Introduction to Ninja Foodi

The traditional pressure cookers evolved impressively with time due to advance technology and tech innovation. Ninja Foodi has raised the bar in the pressure cooker category and has been ranked as one of the most favorite kitchen gadgets of today. The Ninja food is a contemporary pressure cooker integrated with various exclusive features like multi-pressure levels, digital display, timer and a keep warm feature. The most prominent feature that makes Ninja Foodi an extraordinary gadget is that it doubles as an air fryer that not just pressure cooks the food fast but also makes it super crispy. In other words, Ninja Foodi has been developed with Tender Crisp Technology, and can act as multi-use cooker. Mainly, it's a nice blend of air fryer and pressure cooker; however, an inclusion of other important features makes it function beyond that.

How Ninja Foodi Work

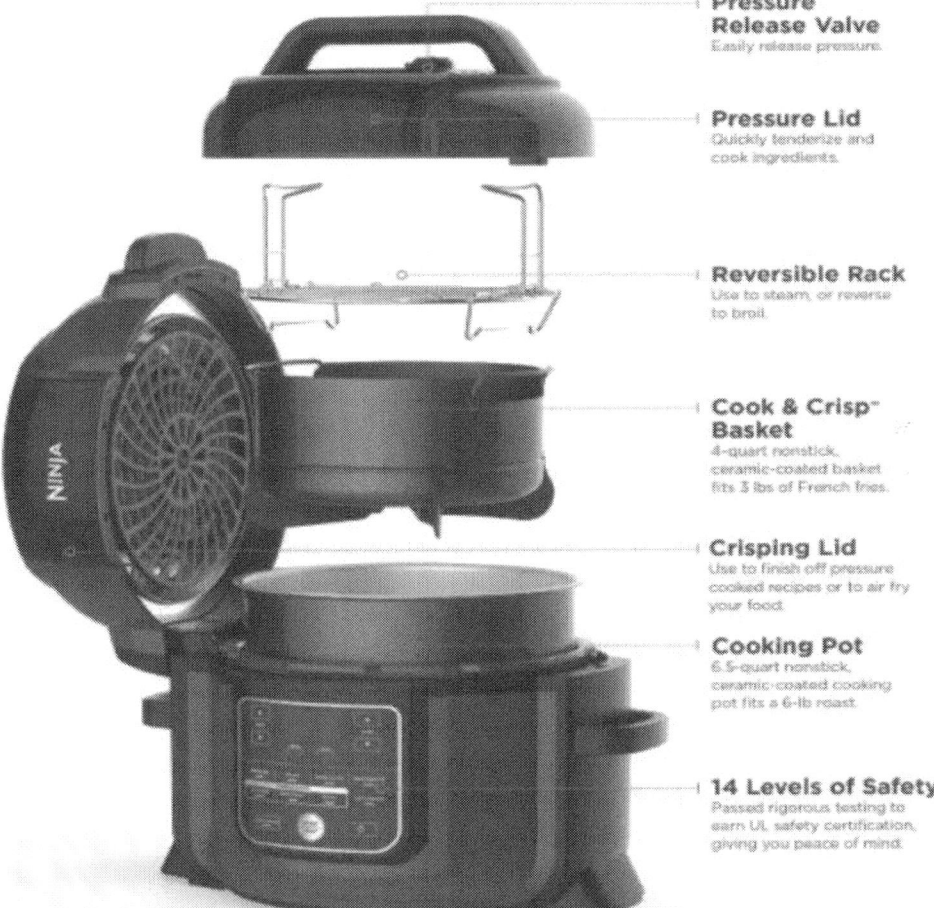

Pressure Release Valve
Easily release pressure.

Pressure Lid
Quickly tenderize and cook ingredients.

Reversible Rack
Use to steam, or reverse to broil.

Cook & Crisp™ Basket
4-quart nonstick, ceramic-coated basket fits 3 lbs of French fries.

Crisping Lid
Use to finish off pressure cooked recipes or to air fry your food.

Cooking Pot
6.5-quart nonstick, ceramic-coated cooking pot fits a 6-lb roast.

14 Levels of Safety
Passed rigorous testing to earn UL safety certification, giving you peace of mind.

The Ninja Foodi is one of the most attractive pressure cookers on the market nowadays. As an electric multi-cooker, it can perform various advanced cooking tasks such as pressure cooking, slow cooking, sautéing, searing, steaming, air frying, broiling, baking, warming, and even dehydrating. This easy-to-use device is designed to cook your food faster and healthier than traditional methods. Essentially, the Ninja Foodi is a sealed pot that creates pressure by heating liquid such as water or stock. In this way, it maintains the steam and constant internal pressure inside the pot. On the other hand, it comes with a cooking basket that allows you to fry your food with less oil. When it comes to the interior, the Ninja

Foodi has a ceramic-coated non-stick cooking pot and Cook & Crisp™ basket. It also comes with five stovetop temperature settings, dual pressure levels (high and low) and a user-friendly control panel that is easy to read. It enables you to set perfect cooking time, temperature and pressure level according to your personal preferences and favorite recipes.

Rules for Using the Ninja Foodi

1. Read a manual before using the product.
2. The Ninja Foodi is equipped with multiple safety features (even 14 levels of safety), but you should always be careful with pressure cookers.
3. Do not touch hot surfaces; always use handles and kitchen gloves.
4. Keep your hands and face away from the steam coming from the vent.
5. Be careful when removing the pressure lid; never force it open.
6. Do not fill the cooking pot beyond the recommended level at 2/3 full (or 1/3 full if you cook rice, grains, legumes, and dried beans).
7. As for pressure cooking, simply put your ingredients into the inner pot. Seal the PRESSURE LID and choose the desired function. Afterwards, release pressure from your cooker.
8. As for air frying, add your ingredients to the cooking basket, use the crisping lid and choose the desired function, time and temperature. Press the START/STOP button.

Function Buttons in Foodi Crisping Pressure

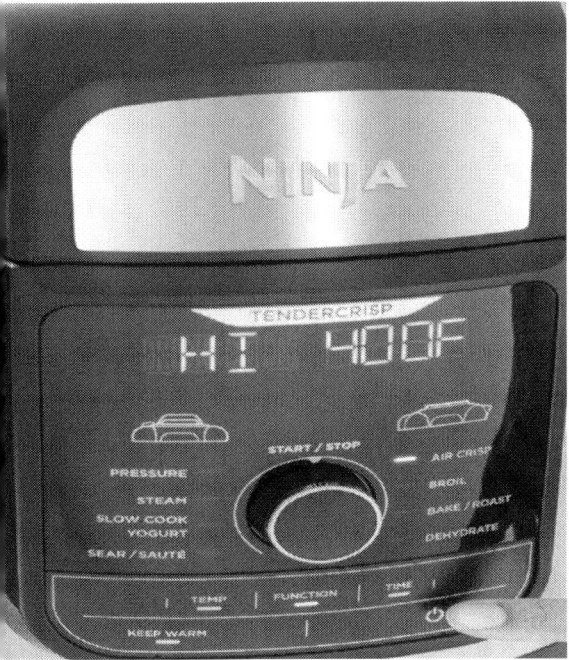

PRESSURE COOK – this is the most common function of your Ninja Foodi. How does it work? Here are basic steps:
1. Lock the pressure lid and turn the valve to seal;
2. Set the time and adjust temperature;
3. Wait for unit to build pressure;
4. When cooking is complete, the unit will beep so you can release the pressure; otherwise, unit will switch to the KEEP WARM function. This is the common function because you can control the time and temperature yourself and customize them according to your recipe or your personal preferences.

STEAM – this is an ideal program for delicate foods such as vegetables and seafood because they require short cooking time, preheated steam, and precise temperature control. You will be able to prepare fresh or frozen foods in less than no time. For instance, beets can be completely steamed in about 15 minutes, cabbage in 3 minutes, and cauliflower will be cooked in 2 minutes. Use a reversible rack that comes with your device in lower position.

SLOW COOK – you can have your dinner ready for when you come back home. Use this program for slow cooking and simmering.

SAUTE/SEAR – go one step further and use this mode to brown meats, sauté vegetables, and thicken the sauces and gravies; cooking on this setting can maximize flavors, too.

AIR CRISP – you can "fry" your favorite food without drenching them in oil. How does it work? Use Cook & Crisp™ basket with this function. You can adjust the temperature between 300 degrees F to 400 degrees F according to your needs. Further, you can open the lid during cooking process to shake the cooking basket or toss ingredients with silicone tipped-tongs for even cooking; when done, put the cooking basket back into the pot and secure the crisping lid. Cooking will automatically resume after that. If you tend to fry smaller chunks that could fall through the rack, you can wrap them in a piece of foil. Use this function to reheat your meals, too.

BAKE/ROAST – this program works as a typical oven; you can make casseroles, frittatas, and desserts. You can choose a temperature between 250 degrees F and 400 degrees F.

BROIL – this program uses intense direct heat to cook food. It provides a caramelizing and charring that give your food that distinct flavor. You do not have to heat your grill or oven to achieve great results in the kitchen – just use a reversible rack in higher position.

DEHYDRATE – you can dehydrate your food in an easy way and have your own dried fruits and vegetables all year long. You can choose the temperature between 105 degrees F and 195 degrees F. Use the Cook & Crisp™ basket and a dehydrating rack.

START/STOP – Use this button to Start or Cancel a function or turn off your Multi-cooker. When you pressure-cooking time is up, it will automatically switch to Keep Warm.

KEEP WARM – once cooking is complete; the unit will automatically switch to this mode and start counting. It will take 12 hours. To keep your food safe, pay attention to food safety temperatures. To prevent your meal from drying out, just leave the lid closed.

TEMP ARROWS: Use the up and down TEMP arrows to adjust the cook temperature and/or pressure level.

TIME ARROWS: Use the up and down TIME arrows to adjust the cook time.

QUICK PRESSURE RELEASE – turn the pressure release valve to the VENT position to release pressure quickly.

NATURAL PRESSURE RELEASE – steam will release from the unit as it cools down. A natural pressure release can take up to 20 minutes, depending on the amount of food. When the pressure is fully released, the red float valve will drop down, so you can remove the lid.

STANDBY MODE: After 10 minutes with no interaction with the control panel, the unit will enter standby mode.

What You Can Do with Ninja Foodi

What can you cook with your Ninja Foodi? The simple answer is – you can cook almost everything in your Ninja Foodi thanks to its tender-crisp technology and multiple functions. Based on the foregoing, we can conclude that there are just so many possibilities.

RICE & GRAINS are extremely versatile. Give your family a new way of enjoying grains! Extremely picky eaters will love rice and grains that are cooked in the cooking pot and then finished off in the cooking basket using the AIR CRISP function. The flavors are infused into rice and grains while cooking in the Ninja Foodi. Before pressure cooking, rinse your grains in a fine mesh strainer under running tap water. After releasing pressure, stir and fluff rice for about 1 minute. You can use PRESSURE button to cook rice and grains fast, while maintaining tenderness. You can cook white rice in 2 to 3 minutes; wild rice will take 22 minutes, while brown rice will take 15 minutes. Further, you can cook polenta in 4 minutes and steel-cut oats in 11 minutes.

BEANS should be soaked 8–12 hours before pressure cooking. Of course, you can cook dried beans without soaking in your Ninja Foodi. It will take about 30 minutes and beans will triple in quantity when cooked. Therefore, for 1 cup of dried beans, you will have 3 cups of cooked beans.

MEATS & POULTRY can be cooked to perfection in your Ninja Foodi. Tough cuts of meat such as chuck roast, flank steak or brisket turn out succulent, juicy and delicious. This will remind you of your grandma's kitchen. Rest the meat for about 5 minutes before slicing in order to seal in the natural juices.

VEGETABLES maintain their authentic flavor. The Ninja Foodi is an amazing one-pot kitchen appliance that uses the latest flavor infusion technology to cook delicious and nutritious vegetable dishes. This advanced technology uses super-heated steam to lock in all the aroma and nutrients in your food. It is almost magic!

FROZEN FOODS. You can put them directly into the cooking pot without defrosting them; just add an extra 10 minutes to the cook time.

How to Use the Foodi Crisping Pressure Cooker

1. **Preparing your ingredients**

Prepare ingredients according to the directions in the pressure-cooking recipe you have selected. For extra flavor, use the brown or sauté functions first, just like you would when cooking with conventional cookware. For instance, brown the meat and vegetables for a stew, before adding other liquids and cooking under pressure. Be sure to deglaze the pot, scraping up any browned bits clinging to the bottom with a small amount of wine, broth or even water, so they loosened, adding flavor to your food, as well as discouraging scorching.

2. **Add Liquid**

After the aromatics softened, add the remaining ingredients and pour liquid, into the cooker body, as specified in the recipe or timetable. This fluid is usually water. However, some recipes will call for other liquids, such as wine.

3. **Lock the lid**

Assemble the pressure lid by aligning the arrow on the front of the lid with the arrow on the front of the cooker base. Then turn the lid clockwise until it locks into place. Make sure the pressure release valve on the lid is in the SEAL position.

4. **Select the function**

Select the function, according to the recipe. Press the START/STOP button to begin. Your Foodi will begin to build pressure, indicated by the rotating lights. The unit will begin counting down when it is fully pressurized

5. **Turn off the cooker and release the pressure.**

When the countdown is finished, the Foodi will beep, automatically switch to the Keep Warm mode, and begin counting up. After the pressure-cooking time has finished, turn off the cooker by selecting "Start/Stop" button. You can release the pressure two ways: quick release and natural release, according to the recipe or timetable instructions.

6. **Air Frying and Finish the dish**

In some cases, after releasing pressure and carefully removing the lid, some dishes need Air fry, bake, roast, or broil to evenly crisp and caramelize meals to golden-brown perfection, finish with a crisp to create Crisp meals or simmer to help thicken, reduce, or concentrate the liquid; others require to add more ingredients to finish the recipe.

Cleaning & Maintenance of Your Foodi Pressure cooker

Cleaning: Dishwasher & Hand-Washing

The unit should be cleaned thoroughly after every use.

1. Unplug the unit from the wall outlet before cleaning.
2. **NEVER** put the cooker base in the dishwasher or immerse it in water or any other liquid.
3. To clean the cooker base and the control panel, wipe them clean with a damp cloth.
4. The cooking pot, silicone ring, reversible rack, Cook & Crisp Basket, and detachable diffuser can be washed in the dishwasher.
5. The pressure lid, including the pressure release valve and anti-clog cap, can be washed with water and dish soap. **DO NOT** wash the pressure lid or any of its components in the dishwasher, and **DO NOT** take apart the pressure release valve or red float valve assembly.
6. To clean the crisping lid, wipe it down with a wet cloth or paper towel after the heat shield cools.
7. If food residue is stuck on the cooking pot, reversible rack, or Cook & Crisp Basket, fill the pot with water and allow to soak before cleaning. **DO NOT** use scouring pads. If scrubbing is necessary, use a non-abrasive cleanser or liquid dish soap with a nylon pad or brush.
8. Air-dry all parts after each use.

Removing & Reinstalling the Silicone Ring

To remove the silicone ring, pull it outward, section by section, from the silicone ring rack. The ring can be installed with either side facing up. To reinstall, press it down into the rack section by section. After use, remove any food debris from the silicone ring and anti-clog cap.

Keep the silicone ring clean to avoid odor.

Washing it in warm, soapy water or in the dishwasher can remove odor. However, it is normal for it to absorb the smell of certain acidic foods. It is recommended to have more than one silicone ring on hand.

NEVER pull out the silicone ring with excessive force, as that may deform it and the rack and affect the pressure-sealing function. A silicone ring with cracks, cuts, or other damage should be replaced immediately.

Useful Tips for Your Foodi Crisping Pressure cooker

1. For consistent browning, make sure ingredients are arranged in an even layer on the bottom of the cooking pot with no overlapping. If ingredients are overlapping, make sure to shake half way through the set cook time.
2. **Watch out about overfilling.** Your Ninja foodi should not be completely filled. Ever! You need space for pressure and/or steam to build up. Whether you are filling it with food or fluid, always make sure there is plenty of space from the top.
3. For smaller ingredients that could fall through the reversible rack, we recommend first wrapping them in a parchment paper or foil pouch.
4. **DO NOT** use a damaged removable cooking pot, silicone ring or lid Replace before using.
5. When switching from pressure cooking to using the crisping lid it is recommended to empty the pot of any remaining liquid for best crisping results.
6. Press and hold down the Time Up or Down arrows to move faster through the display to get to your desired time.

7. **Unplug from outlet when not in use and before cleaning**. Allow to cool before putting on or taking off parts.

8. Use the Keep Warm mode to keep food at a warm, food-safe temperature after cooking. To prevent food from drying out, we recommend keeping the lid closed and using this function just before serving. To reheat food, use the Air Crisp function.

9. **DO NOT** touch hot surfaces. Appliance surfaces are hot during and after operation. To prevent burns or personal injury, ALWAYS use protective hot pads or insulated oven mitts and use available handles and knobs

10. To have your unit build pressure quicker, set it to SEAR/SAUTÉ HIGH. Once ready to pressure cook, press the PRESSURE button and continue as you normally would.

11. **NEVER** use **SLOW COOK** setting without food and liquids in the removable cooking pot.

12. **DO NOT** attempt to open the lid during or after pressure cooking until all internal pressure has been released through the pressure release valve and the unit has cooled slightly. If the lid will not turn to unlock, this indicates the appliance is still under pressure - DO NOT force lid open. Any pressure remaining can be hazardous. Let unit naturally release pressure or turn the Pressure Release Valve to the VENT position to release steam. Take care to avoid contact with the releasing steam to avoid burns or injury. When the steam is completely released, the red float valve will be in the lower position allowing the lid to be removed.

13. **Do not leave the house when it is on**. Unlike with a traditional slow cooker, the Ninja Foodi reaches high temperatures, can carry a high voltage, and involves literal pressure

Ninja Foodi Cook Settings

FUNCTION	Time	Temp
Air Crisp	1-60 minutes	300 to 400
Bake/Roast	1min to 4hr	250 to 400
Broil	1-30 minutes	Auto Set at 450. Not adjustable
Dehydrate	1hr to 12hr	105 to 195
Pressure	1min to 4hr	Lo
		Hi
Steam	10 20 30 min	No temp option
Slow Cook	6hr to 12hr	Lo
		Hi
Sear/Sauté	No time option	Lo
		LOMD
		MD
		MD Hi
		Hi

Foodi Air Crisp Conversion Chart

Type	Food	Crisping Temp	Crisping Lid Time, Fresh	Crisping Lid Time, Frozen	Oil?	Notes
VEGGIES						
	Frozen Hash Browns	350		20 min	Lightly Sprayed	
	Frozen Tater Tots	400		12 min		
	French Fries	400	20 min	400 @15-20 min	Spray	Soak 30 min prior if fresh cut
	Corn on the Cob	360	25 min			Foil Wrapped/Turn 1X
	Roasted Cauliflower	350	15 min		Rub with Oil	Add 1 cup water to bottom
	Green Beans	350	12 min			
	Tomatoes	370	10-12 min			
	Peppers	400	12 min			
	Roasted Asparagus	370	10 min			Preheat 2 min
	Whole Potato	370	35 min			
	Potato, 1/2 length	360	30 min			
	Red Potatoes	350	25 min			Shake a few times
	Potato Wedges	390	16 min		Spray	
	Baked Apples, Cored	360	20 min			Cut in half
BAKING						
	Air Fried Corn Chips	370	5 min		Lightly Sprayed	
	Canned Biscuits	330	6 min			Baking dish
	Frozen Biscuits	350		12 min		Baking dish
	Cake	300	25 min/Foil 10 more			Baking dish
	Quiche	360	20-22 min			Baking dish
	Muffins	390	15-18 min			Baking dish
	Sweet snacks	320	20 min			Baking dish

Foodi Pressure Cooker Chart

Food	Sauté	Time Fresh	Time Frozen	Pressure Level	Opening Method	Opening Time	Notes
Rice/Grain/Oats							
Basmati							1.5 cups water per 1 cup rice
Black Rice		20		High	Slow Normal	10	1.25 cups water per 1 cup rice
Brown Rice		25		High	Slow Normal	10	1.25 cups water per 1 cup rice
Grits		10		High	Quick Release		
Jasmine Rice		1		High	Slow Normal	10	1.25 cups water per 1 cup rice
Oats, Quick		1		High	Slow Normal	10	2 cups water per 1 cup oats
Oats, Rolled		10		High	Natural	20-30	2 cups water per 1 cup oats
Oats, Steel Cut		10		High	Slow Normal	10	3 cups water per 1 cup oats
Pasta		4		High	Normal	3	Cover with water
Quinoa		1		High	Natural	20-30	1.5 cups water per 1 cup quinoa
Risotto		5		High	Slow Normal	10	2 cups water

Wild Rice		20		High	Natural	20-30	1 cup water per 1 cup rice
White Rice		12					1 cup water per 1 cup rice
Veggies							
Asparagus		1		High	Normal	3	
Bell Pepper		4		High	Normal	3	
Black Eyed Peas		7		High	Natural	20-30	
Black Beans		26		High	Natural	20-30	Cover with water
Broccoli		5		High	Normal	3	
Cauliflower Florets		3		High	Normal	3	
Corn on Cob		4		High	Natural	3	
Green Beans		3		High	Normal	3	
Mushrooms		5		High	Normal	3	
Potatoes, baby small		6		High	Normal	3	
Potatoes, Sweet		10		High	Natural	20-30	1 cup water + rack
Potatoes, whole		13		High	Normal	3	1 cup water + rack
Pinto Beans		26		High	Natural	20-30	Cover with water
Veggie Chunks		3		High	Normal	3	1 cup water + rack

Chapter Two: Recipe Conversion Table

Ninja Foodi Cook Settings

FUNCTION	Time	Temp
Air Crisp	1-60 minutes	300 to 400
Bake/Roast	1min to 4hr	250 to 400
Broil	1-30 minutes	Auto Set at 450. Not adjustable
Dehydrate	1hr to 12hr	105 to 195
Pressure	1min to 4hr	Lo
		Hi
Steam	10 20 30 min	No temp option
Slow Cook	6hr to 12hr	Lo
		Hi
Sear/Sauté	No time option	Lo
		LOMD
		MD
		MD Hi
		Hi

Foodi Air Crisp Conversion Chart

Type	Food	Crisping Temp	Crisping Lid Time, Fresh	Crisping Lid Time, Frozen	Oil?	Notes
VEGGIES						
	Frozen Hash Browns	350		20 min	Lightly Sprayed	
	Frozen Tater Tots	400		12 min		
	French Fries	400	20 min	400 @15-20 min	Spray	Soak 30 min prior if fresh cut
	Corn on the Cob	360	25 min			Foil Wrapped/Turn 1X
	Roasted Cauliflower	350	15 min		Rub with Oil	Add 1 cup water to bottom
	Green Beans	350	12 min			
	Tomatoes	370	10-12 min			
	Peppers	400	12 min			
	Roasted Asparagus	370	10 min			Preheat 2 min
	Whole Potato	370	35 min			
	Potato, 1/2 length	360	30 min			
	Red Potatoes	350	25 min			Shake a few times
	Potato Wedges	390	16 min		Spray	
	Baked Apples, Cored	360	20 min			Cut in half
BAKING						
	Air Fried Corn Chips	370	5 min		Lightly Sprayed	
	Canned Biscuits	330	6 min			Baking dish
	Frozen Biscuits	350		12 min		Baking dish
	Cake	300	25 min/Foil 10 more			Baking dish
	Quiche	360	20-22 min			Baking dish
	Muffins	390	15-18 min			Baking dish
	Sweet snacks	320	20 min			Baking dish

Foodi Pressure Cooker Chart

Food	Sauté	Time Fresh	Time Frozen	Pressure Level	Opening Method	Opening Time	Notes
Rice/Grain/Oats							
Basmati							1.5 cups water per 1 cup rice
Black Rice		20		High	Slow Normal	10	1.25 cups water per 1 cup rice
Brown Rice		25		High	Slow Normal	10	1.25 cups water per 1 cup rice
Grits		10		High	Quick Release		
Jasmine Rice		1		High	Slow Normal	10	1.25 cups water per 1 cup rice
Oats, Quick		1		High	Slow Normal	10	2 cups water per 1 cup oats
Oats, Rolled		10		High	Natural	20-30	2 cups water per 1 cup oats
Oats, Steel Cut		10		High	Slow Normal	10	3 cups water per 1 cup oats
Pasta		4		High	Normal	3	Cover with water
Quinoa		1		High	Natural	20-30	1.5 cups water per 1 cup quinoa
Risotto		5		High	Slow Normal	10	2 cups water

Wild Rice	20		High	Natural	20-30	1 cup water per 1 cup rice
White Rice	12					1 cup water per 1 cup rice
Veggies						
Asparagus	1		High	Normal	3	
Bell Pepper	4		High	Normal	3	
Black Eyed Peas	7		High	Natural	20-30	
Black Beans	26		High	Natural	20-30	Cover with water
Broccoli	5		High	Normal	3	
Cauliflower Florets	3		High	Normal	3	
Corn on Cob	4		High	Natural	3	
Green Beans	3		High	Normal	3	
Mushrooms	5		High	Normal	3	
Potatoes, baby small	6		High	Normal	3	
Potatoes, Sweet	10		High	Natural	20-30	1 cup water + rack
Potatoes, whole	13		High	Normal	3	1 cup water + rack
Pinto Beans	26		High	Natural	20-30	Cover with water
Veggie Chunks	3		High	Normal	3	1 cup water + rack

Chapter Three: Introduction to Keto

What is the Ketogenic Diet?

You might have heard your friends talking about ketosis, the Ketogenic diet, etc. And, here you are researching about what they are talking about so passionately. The Ketogenic diet has now become well known for losing weight through a strange phenomenon. It is called strange because for some people depending upon fats for losing fats sounds astonishing! We cannot normally imagine that we have to eat the same thing that we want to eliminate from our body - fats! The Ketogenic diet consists of high amounts of fats, ample proteins and fewer carbohydrates. It forces the body to use fats instead of carbs for breaking down to convert them into energy. In our regular diets, we consume more carbohydrate and shun fats. Thus, our body is perfectly adapted throughout history to break down carbohydrates for energy. However, in the Ketogenic diet, we try to change the pattern of our body to break down the elements to be used for energy. We feed our body with more fats and less carbohydrates and thus force it to adapt in a new way to use fats for energy.

The plus side to this diet is that you do not have to count your calories or the amount of fats you are consuming like the way you do in other diets. You can indulge in different types of meats and oils, do not feel guilty and still lose weight. Normally, our body would convert food into glucose that would be transported to various body parts. This glucose is especially important in fueling functions of the brain. It is easiest for your body to convert carbs into glucose and use it as energy. Thus, it is obvious that your body will choose carbs over any other source of energy. Our body produces insulin to process glucose in the bloodstream and makes it travel around the body. Since glucose is there to provide energy to your body, fats are not required and hence, stored.

However, if you do not feed your body with carbohydrates, the liver starts converting fats to ketone bodies and fatty acids. These ketone bodies enter the brain and pass through it to replace the old source of energy, which was glucose.

Thus, all the fats you consume in the form of meats, oils, creams, etc. is broken down and it does not get accumulated in your body.

When you lower down the carb's intake, the body is persuaded to enter into a state of ketosis. It is just a natural process, which is initiated by the body to help it survive when the food consumption is low. The Ketogenic diet is known by some other names as well- low carbs high fat diet (LCHF), low carb diet. The ultimate aim of a well-maintained Ketogenic diet is to persuade the body into a metabolic state. But this does not mean that you have to go hungry on calories. However, you just have to strictly control your consumption of carbohydrates. It is definitely easier than starving on fats. Human body is extremely adaptive to everything it is forced into. If you make it depend on a new source of energy rather than the regular one, it will adapt accordingly in a few days.

How to Lose Weight with the Ketogenic Diet?

The following tips should be applied while losing weight through the ketogenic diet plan:

1. **Choose a diet containing fewer carbohydrates**

You need to cut down on your consumption of starch and sugar. This idea is more than a century old. There have been a lot of diet plans which are based on reducing the amount of carbs you take. The new thing with the Ketogenic diet is that you provide your body with an alternate source of energy to depend on, which is fats. When you do not eat carbohydrates or eat them moderately, your body is capable of burning 300 additional calories per day, even when you are resting! It means that this amount of burnt calories is equal to a gym session of moderate physical activity.

2. **Eat when you feel hungry**

You do not need to stay hungry all the time to lose weight. This is the most common mistake committed by people who start a low carb diet. In the Ketogenic diet, you do not have to be scared of fats. Carbohydrates and fats are two major sources of energy for our body. If you are snatching carbs from your body, you need to give it an ample supply of fats. Low fats and low carbs equal to starvation, and we do not want that, do we? Starvation results in cravings and fatigue. That is why, people who starve give up easily on their diet plans. The better solution is to consume natural fat till the time you are satisfied. Some of the natural fats are full fat cream, butter, olive oil, meat, bacon, fatty fish, coconut oil, eggs.

3. **Eat real food**

This is one more common mistake made by Ketogenic followers that they get fooled by the fraudulent but creative marketing of "low-carb" foods. A real Ketogenic diet should be supported by real food. It implies the food which is being eaten by humans for millions of years. For example, fish, meat, vegetables, olive oil, butter, nuts, etc.

4. **Eat only if you feel hungry**

You must have read tip number 2 above. In the Ketogenic diet, eat when you are hungry. Do not eat when you are not feeling hungry. Let us elaborate why we are stressing this point again. Unnecessary snacking may become a mammoth issue in the Ketogenic diet. Some products are just so easily available, and they are so tempting that you cannot resist them.

5. **You can skip meals**

Yes, you heard it right. You can even skip breakfast if you are not feeling hungry. This holds truth for any meal. When you are strictly following the Ketogenic diet, your hunger goes down significantly, especially if you have to lose a lot of weight. Your body is happily busy in burning excess fats and reduces your temptation to eat.

6. **Wisely measure your development**

Losing weight successfully might get trickier sometimes. If you focus on your weight all the time and step on the weighing scale all the time, you may get mislead. It de-motivates you and makes you anxious needlessly.

7. **Be persistent**

You would have all those chunks of fats around your waist and thighs in several years. So, how do you expect to lose all the extra fat in just a few weeks? If you want to shed that extra weight permanently, you have to make persistent efforts.

Keto Friendly Foods

Below are some examples of what food you should eat when you're on Ketogenic diet:

Fruits & Vegetables

- Asparagus
- Avocados
- Alfalfa sprouts
- Bell peppers
- Blueberries
- Blackberries
- Broccoli
- Coconut
- Carrot (In moderation)
- Cabbage
- Cranberries
- Cauliflower
- Celery
- Lemon
- Garlic (In moderation)
- Cucumbers
- Chicory
- Green beans
- Jicama
- Herbs
- Mushrooms
- Pumpkin
- Radishes

- Pickles
- Raspberries
- Salad greens
- Scallions
- Zucchini
- Tomatoes
- Strawberries
- Tomatoes
- Spaghetti squash (moderately)
- Okra
- Olives
- Limes
- Onions (In moderation)

Meats & Seafoods
- Crab
- Beef
- Chicken
- Duck
- Goose
- Lamb
- Fish
- Octopus
- Mussels
- Lobsters
- Quail
- Sausage
- Pork
- Shrimp

- Scallops
- Venison
- Veal

Diary

- Cottage cheese
- Burrata cheese
- Blue cheese dressing
- Cream cheese eggs
- Grilling cheese
- Greek yogurt (full-fat)
- Heavy whipping cream
- Halloumi cream
- Homemade whipped cream
- Mozzarella cheese
- Kefalotyri cheese
- Provolone cheese
- Queso blanco
- Ranch dressing
- Ricotta cheese
- Unsweetened almond milk
- Unsweetened coconut milk

Foods to Avoid on Keto Diet
Fruits & Vegetables

- Apricots
- Apples
- Bananas
- Artichokes

Mariana Cleff

- Beans (all varieties)
- Boysenberries
- Butternut squash
- Burdock root
- Cantaloupe
- Cherries
- Chickpeas
- Corn
- Currants
- Edamame
- Egg plants
- Dates
- Elderberries
- Gooseberries
- Grapes
- Mangoes
- Leaks
- Huckleberries
- Honeydew melons
- Kiwifruit
- Parsnips
- Peaches
- Peas
- Potatoes
- Plums
- Pineapples
- Plantains
- Prune

- Raisins
- Taro
- Turnips
- Yams
- Winter squash
- Water chestnuts

Meat and Meats Alternative

- Sausage (with fillers)
- Hot dog (with fillers)
- Seitan
- Tofu
- Deli meat (Some not all)

Diary

- Milk
- Almond milk (sweetened)
- Coconut milk (sweetened)
- Soy milk (regular)
- Yogurt (regular)

Nuts & Seeds

- Pistachios
- Cashew
- Chestnuts

FAQS About Keto Diet

Here are some frequently asked questions about Keto diet.

Should I Count Net Carbs or Total carbs?

There's not a one-size-fits all approach, but what I typically recommend is counting net carbs for vegetables but total carbs for everything else. This recommendation is made because not all carbs are created equal, and some, like green vegetables should be include in your keto lifestyle. However, I don't encourage the consumption of other low-net-carbs processed foods like low-carb tortillas or Atkins bars.

What Should My Macronutrients be?

The macronutrient breakdown is typically 65 to 75 percent fat, 15 to 30 percent protein, and 5 to 10 percent carbohydrates. However, how this translates into grams of proteins carbohydrates and fats needs to be individualized for your body and your goals. I recommend counting macronutrients, especially in the beginning, to learn how best to formulate your diet. There are several online macro calculators that can be used at beginning.

Can I eat Too Much Fat?

Yes, you can definitely eat too much fat, and that is why it is important to follow an individualized macro breakdown. If your goal is fat loss, I recommend only eating fat until satiety. When following a keto lifestyle, your body's main fuel source will be fat, and this can come dietary fat or body fat. Your body will burn dietary fats first, because it is more readily available. If you are overeating dietary fat, you are giving your body no reason to burn body fat. Eating enough fat is good but overeating fat will not result in fat loss.

Do Calories Matter on a Keto Diet?

Yes, while there is more to fat loss and body recomposition than calories in versus calories out, calories do still matter. Eating too few or eating too many will prevent you from seeing results. Bothe the number of calories you eat and the types of foods that make up those calories will factor into you seeing results. Both the number of calories you eat and the types of foods that make up those calories will factor into you seeing results.

Can I substitute one cut of meat for Another-pork loin For Pork shoulder, for instance, or chicken breasts for chicken thighs?

Different meats have varying amount of connective tissue and fat, which means that they cook at different rates. Substituting one for another is usually possible. It just requires a shorter or longer cooking time.

Chapter Four: Keto Ninja Foodi Breakfast Recipes

Tomato Cups

Servings: 4

Preparation Time: 8 minutes

Ingredients:

- 4 big tomatoes
- 4 eggs
- 7 ounces ham
- 1 tablespoon chives
- 1 teaspoon mayonnaise
- ½ teaspoon butter
- 4 ounces Parmesan cheese
- ½ teaspoon salt

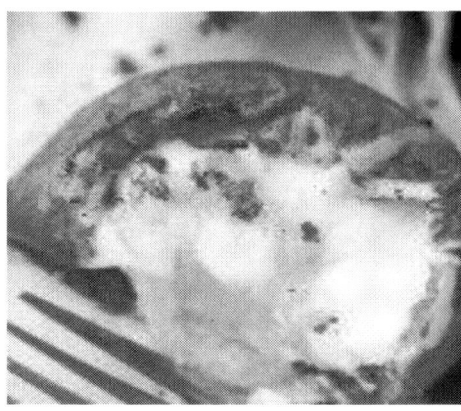

Directions:

1. Wash the tomatoes and remove the flesh, jelly, and seeds from them and add to a mixing bowl. Chop the ham and chives.
2. Combine the chopped ham, chives, and tomato pieces together in a mixing bowl.
3. Add mayonnaise, butter, and salt to the ham mixture and blend well. Grate the Parmesan cheese and beat the eggs in the empty tomato cups. Fill the cups with the ham mixture.
4. Sprinkle them with the grated cheese. Wrap the tomato cups in aluminum foil and transfer them in the pressure cooker.
5. Close the lid, and set the pressure cooker mode to "Sauté." Cook for 10 minutes. When the cooking time ends, remove the tomatoes from the pressure cooker and allow them to rest.

6. Discard the foil and serve immediately.

Nutritional Information: Calories: 335, Fat: 19.8g, Carbohydrates: 12.17g, Protein: 27g

Savory Cheese and Ham Custard

Servings: 4

Preparation Time: 35 minutes

Ingredients:

- 2 serrano ham slices, chopped
- 4 large eggs
- ½ cup cottage cheese, room temperature
- ¼ cup half and half
- Salt and white pepper to taste
- ¼ cup grated Monterey Jack cheese
- ¼ cup caramelized white onions

Directions

1. Select Sear/Sauté mode, adjust to Medium, and choose Start/Stop to preheat the pot for 5 minutes. Cook the ham in the inner pot until brown and crispy, 5 minutes.
2. Transfer to a paper towel-lined plate and set aside. Using a brush, coat the inner parts of four medium ramekins with the ham fat and set aside.
3. Remove and clean the inner pot and return to the base. Crack the eggs into a medium bowl and whisk in the cottage cheese, half and half, salt, and white pepper until no cheese lumps remain.
4. Mix in the Monterey Jack cheese until well-incorporated.
5. Divide the ham in the bottom of each ramekin, top with the onions, and pour in the egg mixture two-thirds way up.
6. Cover each cup with foil.
7. Pour 1 cup of water into the inner pot, fix in the Reversible Rack in the lower position, and arrange the ramekins on top. You may fit three ramekins closely and place the last ramekin in the middle of the three combined ones.

8. Cover with the Pressure Lid and lock the vent to Seal. Select Pressure, adjust to High, and set the timer to 7 minutes.
9. Press Start/Stop to begin cooking. After cooking, perform a quick pressure release to let out all the steam, and open the Pressure Lid.
10. Use tongs to remove the ramekins onto a flat surface, take of the foil and cool for 1 to 2 minutes.
11. Serve afterwards.

Nutritional Information: Calories: 335, Fat: 19.8g, Carbohydrates: 12.17g, Protein: 27g

Keto egg bites

Servings: 4

Preparation Time: 27 minutes

Ingredients

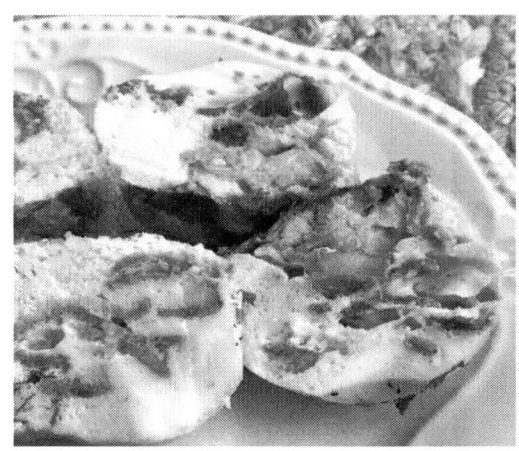

- 4-5 slices of bacon
- 1/2 cup lite coconut milk
- 1 cup Spinach cut up
- 6 eggs
- 4-5 slices of bacon
- 1/2 cup lite coconut milk or regular milk canned

Directions

1. First cook your bacon in the Ninja Foodi. Use your Air crisper basket and placed my slices of bacon inside the basket so that the drippings would land in the ceramic liner.
2. Set at 400 degrees, air crisp for 10 minutes for crispy. Less time if you don't like it crispy
3. Remove crisping basket and set aside.
4. Crack 6 eggs in a mixing bowl, add bacon grease, or omit, it doesn't matter, add spinach, and coconut milk. Salt and pepper to taste if you desire. Mix well.
5. Spray egg bite molds with non-stick butter spray evenly. Set mold on trivet.
6. Pour each mold evenly of mixture. Set trivet and mold in Ninja Foodi. Lower the crisping lid and set at 325 for 17 minutes.
7. Remove and set to cool. Pop out of mold and enjoy with tomato or avocado on top. You may leave eggs in mold and set lid on and place in the fridge for a grab and go snack or breakfast. Yes, these are great cold too!

Veggie Frittata

Servings: 6

Preparation Time: 25 minutes

Ingredients:

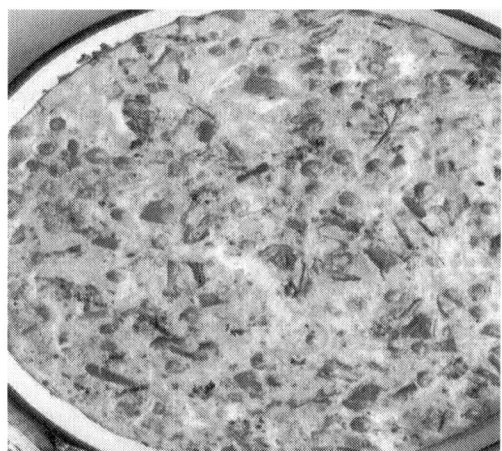

- 10 eggs
- 1 cup of coconut milk
- 1 teaspoon salt
- ½ teaspoon ground black pepper
- 1 sweet bell pepper
- ½ jalapeno pepper
- 3 tomatoes
- 1 zucchini
- 1 tablespoon butter
- 5 ounces asparagus
- ½ cup cilantro

Directions:

1. Beat the eggs in the mixing bowl until combined. Add the coconut milk and butter and combine.
2. Sprinkle the mixture with the salt and, ground black pepper and mix well. Chop the zucchini, tomatoes, asparagus, and cilantro.
3. Remove the seeds from the bell pepper and chop it. Slice the jalapeno pepper. Transfer the egg mixture to the pressure cooker. Top with the vegetables and cilantro.
4. Close the lid, and set the pressure cooker mode to "Steam." Cook for 15 minutes.
5. Remove the frittata from the pressure cooker.
6. Serve immediately.

Nutritional Information: Calories: 145, Fat: 11.4g, Carbohydrates: 5.4g, Protein: 7.1g

Pumpkin Spice Breakfast Cake

Servings: 6

Preparation Time: 40 minutes

Ingredients:

- 8 Tbsp butter
- ½ cup Baking Stevia
- 1 egg
- 1 tsp vanilla
- 2 cups almond flour
- 2 tsp baking powder
- 1 tsp salt
- 1 tsp cinnamon
- ¼ tsp nutmeg
- ¼ tsp ginger
- 1 cup pumpkin puree

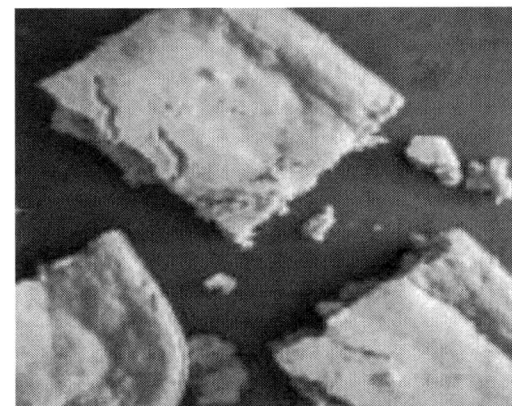

Directions:

1. Use an electric mixer to cream the butter and stevia together until they are light and fluffy.
2. Mix the vanilla and eggs in a small bowl then add to the mixer with the butter blend. Ix until just combined
3. Add the remaining dry ingredients to the mixer and fold together by hand. Add the pumpkin puree and mix until smooth.
4. Pour the cake batter into your Ninja Foodi and place the lid on. Press the air crisp button and set the temperature to 350 degrees and program the timer to 25 minutes. Once cooked, a toothpick should come out of the center of the cake cleanly. Allow to cool and serve.

Nutritional Info (per serving): Calories: 176, Fat: 16g, Carbohydrates: 8g, Protein: 3g

Zucchini Egg Cups

Servings: 4

Preparation Time: 15 minutes

Ingredients:

- 1 zucchini
- 2 tablespoon almond flour
- ½ teaspoon salt
- 1 teaspoon butter
- 4 eggs

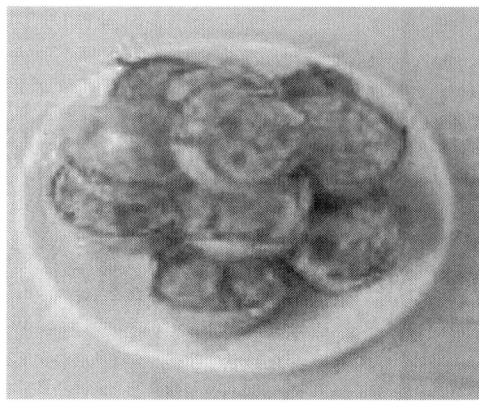

Directions

1. Grate zucchini and mix it up with almond flour and salt.
2. Spread the muffin molds with butter and place grated zucchini inside in the shape of nests. Then beat eggs inside "zucchini nests" and place them in the cooker.
3. Lower the air fryer lid. Cook the zucchini cups for 7 minutes.
4. When the eggs are solid, the meal is cooked.

Nutritional Information: Calories: 99g, Fat: 7.2g, Carbohydrates: 2.7g, Protein: 6.9g

Parmesan Chicken Wings

Servings: 2

Preparation Time: 27 minutes

Ingredients:

- 4 chicken wings
- ½ cup chicken stock
- ½ teaspoon salt
- 1 tablespoon butter, softened
- 1 oz. Parmesan Cheese, grated
- 1 teaspoon garlic powder
- 1 teaspoon minced garlic
- 1 teaspoon dried dill

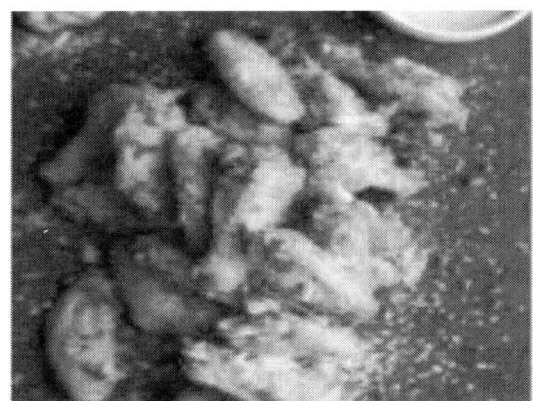

Directions

1. Rub the chicken wings with the salt and place in the Ninja Foodi pot.
2. Add chicken stock and close the lid. Seal the lid and cook chicken wings at Pressure Cook mode (High pressure) for 9 minutes.
3. Meanwhile, mix up together the butter, grated cheese, minced garlic, garlic powder, and dried dill. Whisk the mixture until homogenous.
4. When the chicken wings are cooked – make a quick pressure release. Open the lid and transfer chicken wings on the plate.
5. Remove the liquid from the pot and insert rack.
6. Brush the chicken wings with the butter mixture generously and transfer on the rack.
7. Lower the air fryer lid and press the "Broil" mode. Cook the wings for 8 minutes.
8. Enjoy!

Nutritional Information: Calories: 192g, Fat: 12.4g, Carbohydrates: 2.4g, Protein: 18g

Feta Frittata

Servings: 3

Preparation Time: 25 minutes

Ingredients:

- 4 oz fresh spinach, chopped
- 3 eggs, beaten
- 1 oz Feta, crumbled
- ¼ teaspoon white pepper
- ¼ teaspoon salt

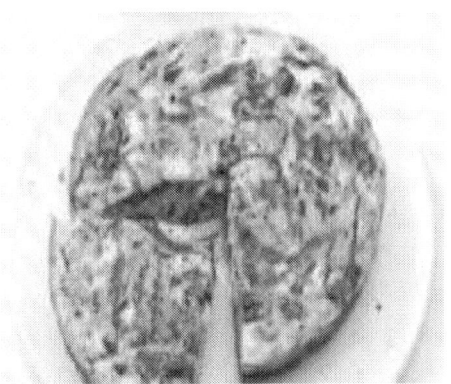

Directions

1. Whisk the eggs well.
2. Stir the spinach in the whisked eggs and add white pepper and salt. After this, add Feta cheese and mix up the egg mixture with the help of the spoon gently
3. Transfer the liquid in the springform pan. Insert the air fryer rack in Ninja Foodi and place the frittata.
4. Lower the air fryer lid and cook frittata at 360 F.
5. Cook for 15 minutes or until the meal is set.
6. Serve!

Nutritional Information: Calories: 97, Fat: 6.5g, Carbohydrates: 2.2g, Protein: 8g

Pancetta Hash with Baked Eggs

Servings: 4

Preparation Time: 60 minutes

Ingredients

- 6 slices pancetta, chopped
- 1 white onion, diced
- 2 turnips, peeled and diced
- 1 tsp sweet paprika
- Salt and freshly ground black pepper to taste
- 1 tsp garlic powder
- 4 eggs

Directions

1. Select Sear/Sauté mode, adjust to Medium High, and choose Start/Stop to preheat the pot for 5 minutes.
2. Once heated, pour the pancetta into the inner pot, and cook with occasional stirring until brown and crispy, 5 minutes.
3. Stir in the onion, turnips, paprika, salt, black pepper, and garlic powder. Close the Air Crisping Lid; choose Bake/Roast, set the temperature to 350°F, and the time to 25 minutes.
4. Cook until the turnips are golden brown and soft while occasionally stirring. Open the lid and crack in the eggs. Close the Air Crisping Lid again, select Bake/Roast mode, temperature to 350°F, and the time to 10 minutes.
5. Cook the eggs and check after 2 to 3 minutes to ensure that they are of your desired cook.
6. Spoon the food into serving bowls and enjoy warm

Nutritional Information: Calories: 146, Fat: 6.93g, Carbohydrates: 8.64g, Protein: 12.21g

Avocado Bacon Bombs

Servings: 4

Preparation Time: 20 minutes

Ingredients:

- 1 avocado, peeled, cored
- 4 oz bacon, sliced
- 1 tablespoon almond flour
- 1 tablespoon flax meal
- ½ teaspoon salt

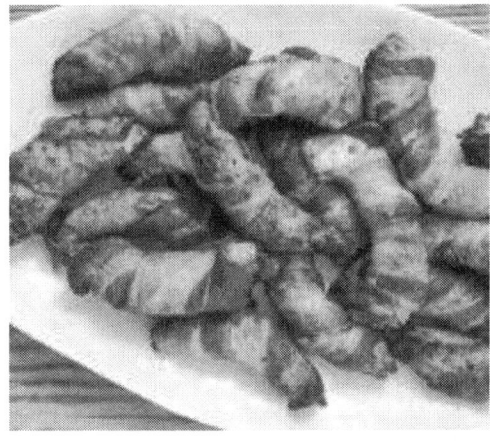

Directions:

1. Blend together avocado, almond flour, flax meal, and salt. When the mixture is smooth, transfer it in the mixing bowl.
2. Make the medium size balls from it and wrap in the bacon.
3. Secure the balls with the toothpicks.
4. After this, transfer the bombs in the cooker and ser air crisp mode. Close the lid and cook the meal for 10 minutes.

Nutritional Information: Calories: 303, Fat: 25.5g, Carbohydrates: 6.7g, Protein: 13.3g

Tortilla Ham Wraps

Serving: 5

Preparation time: 20 minutes

Ingredients:

- 5 almond flour tortillas
- 10 ounces ham
- 2 tomatoes
- 1 cucumber
- 1 red onion
- 1 tablespoon mayonnaise
- 2 tablespoons olive oil
- 2 tablespoons ketchup
- 1 teaspoon basil
- 1 teaspoon paprika
- ½ teaspoon cayenne pepper
- 4 ounces lettuce

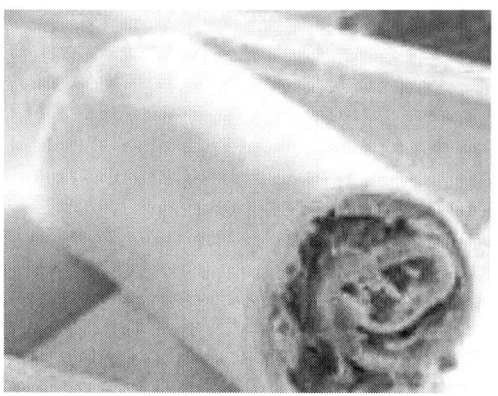

Directions:

1. Slice the tomatoes and chop the cucumbers. Chop the ham.
2. Peel the red onion and chop it. Combine the mayonnaise, olive oil, ketchup, basil, paprika, and cayenne pepper and stir the mixture.
3. Spread the tortillas with the mayonnaise mixture and add chopped ham. Sprinkle the dish with the chopped onion, sliced tomatoes, and chopped cucumbers.
4. Add lettuce and wrap the tortillas. Transfer the tortilla wraps in the pressure cooker and close the lid. Set the pressure cooker mode at "Steam," and cook for 10 minutes.
5. Remove the dish from the pressure cooker and rest briefly.

Nutritional Information: Calories: 249, Fat: 15g, Carbohydrates: 14.7g, Protein: 15.6g

Raspberry Breakfast Cake

Servings: 6

Preparation Time: 40 minutes

Ingredients:

- 8 Tbsp butter
- ½ cup Baking Stevia
- 1 egg
- 1 tsp vanilla
- 2 cups almond flour
- 2 tsp baking powder
- 1 tsp salt
- 1 cup fresh raspberries
- ½ cup buttermilk

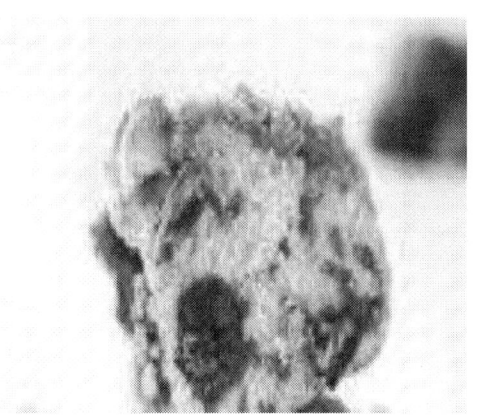

Directions:

1. Use an electric mixer to cream the butter and stevia together until they are light and fluffy.
2. Mix the vanilla and eggs in a small bowl then add to the mixer with the butter blend. Mix until just combined
3. In a separate bowl, toss the raspberries and ¼ cup almond flour to coat the berries.
4. Add the remaining dry ingredients to the mixer and fold together by hand. Add the buttermilk and mix until smooth.
5. Add the raspberries to the batter and mix briefly. Pour the cake batter into your Ninja Foodi and place the lid on.
6. Press the air crisp button and set the temperature to 350 degrees and program the timer to 25 minutes.
7. Once cooked, a toothpick should come out of the center of the cake cleanly. Allow to cool and serve.

Nutritional Info (per serving): Calories: 183g, Fat: 16g, Carbohydrates: 8g, Protein: 3g

Cauliflower Hash browns

Servings: 6

Preparation Time: 35 minutes

Ingredients:

- 6 eggs
- 4 cups riced cauliflower
- ¼ cup milk
- 1 onion, chopped
- 3 Tbsp butter
- 1 ½ cups chopped, cooked ham
- ½ cup shredded cheese

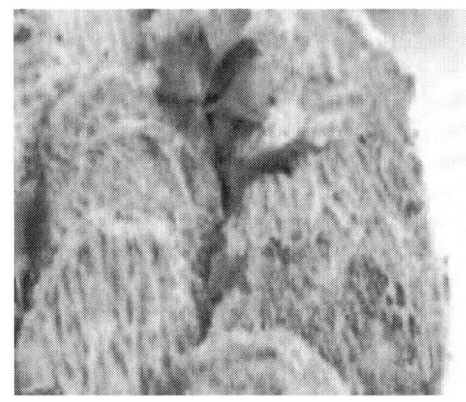

Directions:

1. Press the sauté button on your Ninja Foodi and add the butter and the onions.
2. Cook, stirring occasionally until the onions are soft, about 5 minutes.
3. Add the iced cauliflower to the pot and stir. Turn on the air crisper for 15 minutes, turning the cauliflower halfway through.
4. In a small bowl, mix the eggs and milk together then pour over the browned cauliflower. Sprinkle the ham over the top of the egg mix.
5. Press the air crisp button again and set the timer for 10 minutes.
6. Sprinkle the cheddar cheese on top and close the lid of the Ninja Foodi for one minute to just melt the cheese. Serve while hot

Nutritional Info (per serving): Calories: 166g, Fat: 14g, Carbohydrates: 3g, Protein: 9g

Egg Crumpet Sandwiches

Servings: 4

Preparation Time: 20 minutes

Ingredients:

- 2 tbsp unsalted butter, divided
- 2 bacon slices, chopped
- 4 large eggs
- Salt and freshly ground black pepper to taste
- 2 tbsp grated cheddar cheese
- 4 low carb crumpets, splitted

Directions

1. Brush four medium ramekins with 1 tbsp of butter and divide the bacon into the cups.
2. Crack an egg on each and use a toothpick to prick the eggs.
3. Season with salt, black pepper, and divide the cheddar cheese on top.
4. Cover the ramekins with foil. Pour 1 cup of water into the inner pot, fix in the Reversible Rack in the bottom position, and place the cups on top.
5. Cover with the Pressure Lid and lock the vent to Seal. Select Pressure; adjust to High, and set the cook time to 1 minute. Press Start to begin cooking.
6. After cooking, perform a quick pressure release, and open the lid. Carefully remove the cups, rack, and foil. Empty the inner pot and return to the base.
7. Fix in the Reversible Rack in the upper position and place the ramekins on top. Cover the Air Crisping Lid, select Broil and set the time to 2 minutes.
8. Press Start to begin cooking. Meanwhile, spread the remaining butter in the crumpet halves. Open the Air Crisping Lid, arrange the crumpet halves on the rack with the buttered-side up, and close the lid.
9. Choose Broil again and adjust the cooking time to 4 minutes. Press Start to begin toasting.

10. When the crumpets are ready, transfer to a serving plate, and remove the cups using tongs.
11. Run a butter knife in and around the cups and invert each baked egg onto the lower half of each crumpet. Top with the other half of the crumpets and serve immediately.

Nutritional Information: Calories: 166g, Fat: 14g, Carbohydrates: 3g, Protein: 9g

Cheesy Chorizo Topping

Servings: 6

Preparation Time: 18 minutes

Ingredients:

- 8 ounces chorizo
- ⅓ cup tomato juice
- 1 teaspoon cilantro
- 1 tablespoon coconut flour
- 1 teaspoon olive oil
- 1 teaspoon butter
- 1 sweet bell peppers
- 3 eggs
- ⅓ cup of coconut milk
- 1 teaspoon coriander
- ¼ teaspoon thyme
- ⅓ cup fresh basil

Directions:

1. Combine the tomato juice, cilantro, coconut flour, olive oil, coriander, and thyme.
2. Stir the mixture well. Remove the seeds from the bell peppers and chop it. Wash the fresh basil and chop it.
3. Add coconut milk in the tomato juice mixture and beat the eggs. Blend the mixture using a hand mixer until smooth.
4. Add the chopped peppers and butter. Chop the chorizo and add to the mixture.
5. Transfer the mixture to the pressure cooker and close the lid. Set the pressure cooker mode to "Steam," and cook for 6 minutes. Open the lid and blend well carefully using a wooden spoon.

6. Close the pressure cooker lid, and cook for 2 minutes. When the cooking time ends, let the dish rest briefly. Serve it immediately.

Nutritional Information: Calories: 260g, Fat: 21.4g, Carbohydrates: 4.6g, Protein: 12.7g

Spinach Muffins

Servings: 5

Preparation Time: 28 minutes

Ingredients:

- 2 cup spinach, chopped
- 5 eggs, whisked
- 1 tablespoon flax meal
- ½ teaspoon salt
- 1 teaspoon turmeric
- ½ teaspoon butter
- 1 cup water, for cooking

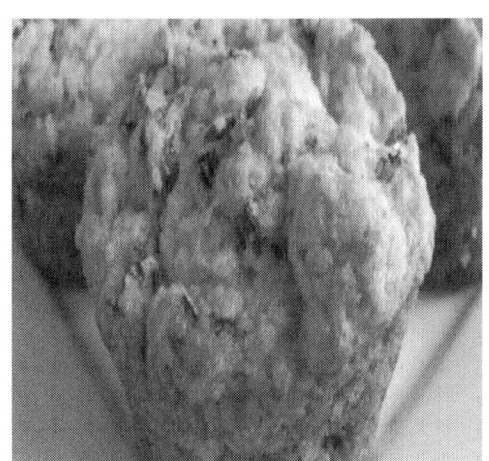

Directions:

1. In the mixing bowl mix up together chopped spinach, whisked eggs, flax meal, salt, turmeric, and butter.
2. Transfer the mixture into the muffin molds. Pour water in the cooker and insert trivet.
3. Place muffin molds on the trivet and close the lid. Cook muffins for 8 minutes on High-pressure mode. Then use quick pressure release.
4. Chill the muffins until warm and remove from the muffin molds.

Nutritional Information: Calories: 77, Fat: 5.3g, Carbohydrates: 1.5g, Protein: 6.7g

Bacon and Egg Bites

Servings: 6

Preparation Time: 30 minutes

Ingredients:

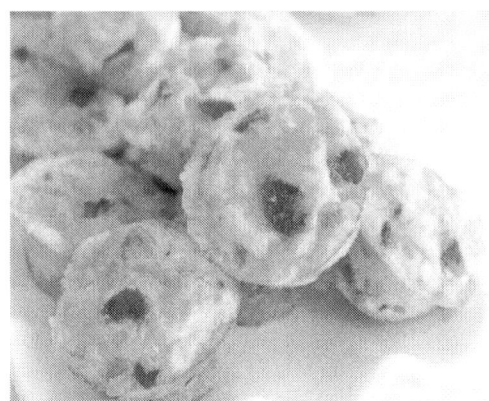

- 5 slices bacon
- ½ cup milk
- 1 cup chopped spinach
- 6 eggs

Directions

1. Place the bacon strips in the Ninja Foodi air crisper basket and use the air crisp function, set for 10 minutes to cook the bacon.
2. Remove the basket and the strips and pour the bacon grease into a separate small bowl.
3. Add the eggs to the bacon grease along with the spinach, crumbled cooked bacon and milk. Spray an egg bite mold and pour the egg mix evenly into each mold.
4. Place the mold on top of the metal trivet inside the Ninja Foodi. Lower the crisper lid and set the temperature for 375 for 17 minutes. Once cooked, remove the egg mold from the Ninja Foodi and let cool. Pop the egg bites out of the mold and serve hot or cold.

Nutritional Info (per serving): Calories: 118g, Fat: 8g, Carbohydrates: 2g, Protein: 9g

Mason Jar Omelet

Servings: 6

Preparation Time: 17 minutes

Ingredients:

- 4 eggs, whisked
- ¼ cup cream
- ½ teaspoon salt
- 2 oz bacon, chopped
- 1 teaspoon butter, melted
- 1 cup water, for cooking

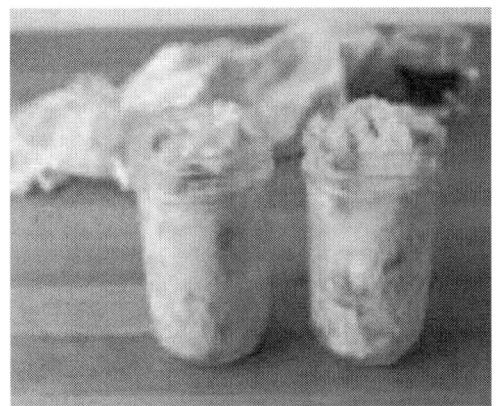

Directions:

1. Mix up together whisked eggs, cream, salt, and chopped bacon. Add melted butter and stir the mixture.
2. Pour egg mixture in the mason jars. Pour 1 cup of water in the Pressure cooker and insert trivet. Place mason jars on the trivet.
3. Close the lid and cook an omelet for 7 minutes on High-pressure mode. Then use quick pressure release. Chill the meal little before serving.

Nutritional Information: Calories: 234g, Fat: 18g, Carbohydrates: 1.2g, Protein: 16.2g

Cinnamon Chia Pudding

Servings: 4

Preparation Time: 25 minutes

Ingredients:

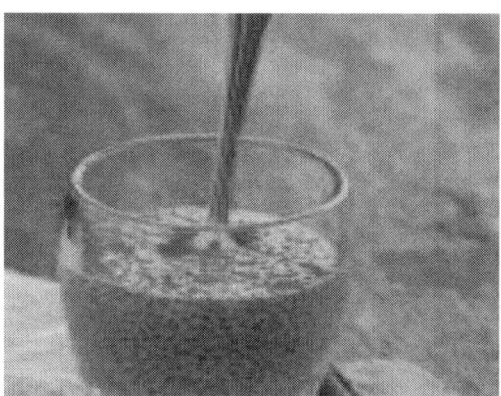

- 1 cup chia seeds
- 4 tablespoons Erythritol
- 2 cups of coconut milk
- 2 tablespoons heavy cream
- 1 teaspoon butter
- 1 teaspoon cinnamon
- 1 teaspoon ground cardamom

Directions:

1. Combine the chia seeds, Erythritol, and coconut milk together in the pressure cooker.
2. Stir the mixture gently and close the lid. Set the pressure cooker mode to "Slow Cook," and cook for 10 minutes.
3. When the cooking time ends, let the chia seeds rest little. Open the pressure cooker lid and add cream, cinnamon, cardamom, and butter.
4. Blend the mixture well using a wooden spoon. Transfer the pudding to the serving bowls.

Nutritional Information: Calories: 486g, **Fat:** 43.4g, **Carbohydrates:** 22.6g, **Protein:** 8.8g

Veggie Egg Casserole

Servings: 4

Preparation Time: 13minutes

Ingredients:

- 4 eggs
- 1 Tbsp milk
- 1 tomato, diced
- ½ cup spinach
- ¼ tsp salt
- ¼ tsp ground black pepper

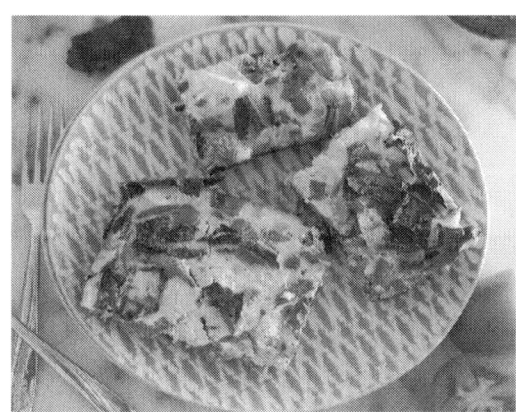

Directions:

1. Prepare a baking pan that fits in your Ninja Foodi bowl by greasing the pan with butter. Set aside
2. In a medium bowl, whisk together the eggs, milk, salt and pepper and then add the veggies to the bowl and stir briefly.
3. Pour the egg mix into the prepared baking pan and lower the pan into the Ninja Foodi. Set the Ninja Foodi to air crisp at 325 for 7 minutes.
4. Remove the pan of eggs from the Ninja Foodi and enjoy while hot!

Nutritional Info (per serving): Calories: 78g, Fat: 5g, Carbohydrates: 1g, Protein: 7g

Ham and Eggs Casserole

Servings: 4

Preparation Time: 13 minutes

Ingredients:

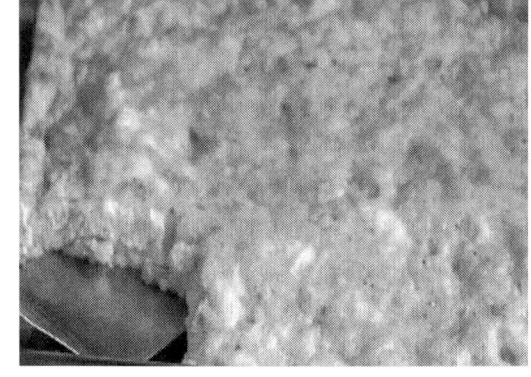

- 4 eggs
- 1 Tbsp milk
- 1 cup cooked, chopped ham
- ½ cup Shredded cheddar cheese
- ¼ tsp salt
- ¼ tsp ground black pepper

Directions:

1. Prepare a baking pan that fits in your Ninja Foodi bowl by greasing the pan with butter. Set aside
2. In a medium bowl, whisk together the eggs, milk, salt and pepper and then add the ham and cheese to the bowl and stir briefly.
3. Pour the egg mix into the prepared baking pan and lower the pan into the Ninja Foodi. Set the Ninja Foodi to air crisp at 325 for 7 minutes.
4. Remove the pan of eggs from the Ninja Foodi and enjoy while hot!

Nutritional Info (per serving): Calories: 169, Fat: 13g, Carbohydrates: 1g, Protein: 12g

Fish with Sesame

Servings: 4

Preparation Time: 16 minutes

Ingredients:

- 1.5-pound salmon fillet
- 1 tablespoon apple cider vinegar
- 1 teaspoon sesame seeds
- ¼ teaspoon dried rosemary
- ½ teaspoon salt
- 1 teaspoon butter, melted

Directions

1. Sprinkle the salmon fillet with the apple cider vinegar.
2. After this, mix up together the sesame seeds, dried rosemary, salt, and butter.
3. Brush the salmon with the butter sauce generously.
4. Place the salmon on the rack and lower the air fryer lid.
5. Set the air fryer mode and cook fish at 360 F for 8 minutes.
6. Serve it!

Nutritional Information: Calories: 239, Fat: 11.8g, Carbohydrates: 0.3g, Protein: 33.1g

Delightful Cheese Casserole

Servings: 8

Preparation Time: 30 minutes

Ingredients:

- 6 ounces cheddar cheese
- 1 zucchini
- ½ cup ground chicken
- 4 ounces Parmesan cheese
- 3 tablespoons butter
- 1 teaspoon paprika
- 1 teaspoon salt
- 1 teaspoon basil
- 1 teaspoon cilantro
- ½ cup fresh dill
- ⅓ cup tomato juice
- ½ cup cream
- 2 red sweet bell peppers

Directions:

1. Grate cheddar cheese. Chop the zucchini and combine it with the ground chicken.
2. Sprinkle the mixture with the paprika, salt, basil, cilantro, tomato juice, and cream. Stir the mixture well.
3. Transfer it to the pressure cooker. Chop the dill, sprinkle the mixture in the pressure cooker, and add the butter. Chop the Parmesan cheese and add it to the pressure cooker.
4. Chop the bell peppers and add them too.
5. Sprinkle the mixture with the grated cheddar cheese and close the lid.

6. Set the pressure cooker mode to "Sauté", and cook for 30 minutes. When the cooking time ends, let the casserole chill briefly and serve.

Nutritional Information: Calories: 199, Fat: 14.7g, Carbohydrates: 6.55g, Protein: 11g

Bacon, Broccoli and Cheddar Frittata

Servings: 4

Preparation Time: 12 minutes

Ingredients:

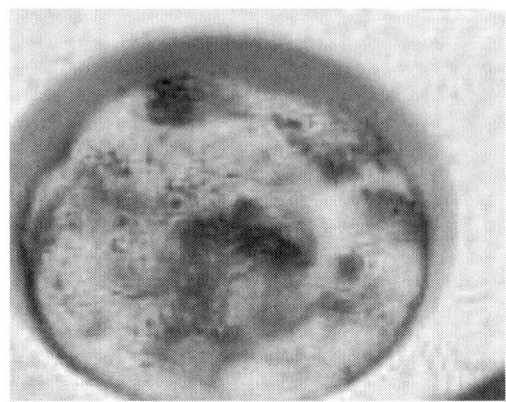

- 6 eggs
- 2 Tbsp milk
- ½ cup chopped, cooked bacon
- 1 cup cooked broccoli
- ½ cup shredded cheddar cheese
- ¼ tsp salt
- ¼ tsp ground black pepper

Directions:

1. Prepare a baking pan that fits in your Ninja Foodi bowl by greasing the pan with butter. Set aside
2. In a medium bowl, whisk together the eggs, milk, salt and pepper and then add the bacon, broccoli and cheese to the bowl and stir briefly.
3. Pour the egg mix into the prepared baking pan and lower the pan into the Ninja Foodi. Set the Ninja Foodi to air crisp at 325 for 7 minutes.
4. Remove the pan of eggs from the Ninja Foodi and enjoy while hot

Nutritional Info (per serving): Calories: 269, Fat: 20g, Carbohydrates: 3g, Protein: 19g

Coconut Oatmeal

Servings: 6

Prep Time: 25 minutes

Ingredients:

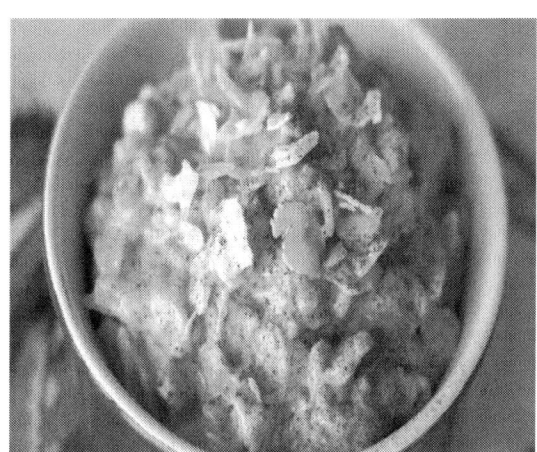

- 1 cup shredded dried coconut flakes
- 3 cups coconut milk
- 3 cups water
- ¼ cup psyllium husks
- ½ cup coconut flour
- 1 ½ tsp vanilla extract
- ½ tsp cinnamon
- ½ cup granulated stevia

Directions:
1. Add all of the ingredients into the Ninja Foodi and stir together briefly
2. Place the lid on and set the steamer valve to seal. Set the pressure cooker function to 1 minute (it will take about 10 minutes to come to pressure). When the oatmeal is done, do a quick pressure release by opening the steamer valve carefully. Serve while hot

Nutritional Information: Calories: 202, Fat: 16g, Carbohydrates: 6g, Protein: 3g

Spicy Bacon Bites

Servings: 8

Preparation Time: 26 minutes

Ingredients:

- 10 ounces Romano cheese
- 6 ounces sliced bacon
- 1 teaspoon oregano
- 5 ounces puff pastry
- 1 teaspoon butter
- 2 egg yolks
- 1 teaspoon sesame seeds

Directions:

1. Chop Romano cheese into small cubes. Roll the puff pastry using a rolling pin. Whisk the egg yolks. Sprinkle them with the oregano and sesame seeds.
2. Cut the puff pastry into the squares, and place an equal amount of butter on every square. Wrap the cheese cubes in the sliced bacon.
3. Place the wrapped cheese cubes onto the puff pastry squares. Make the "bites" of the dough and brush them with the egg yolk mixture.
4. Transfer the bites in the pressure cooker. Close the lid, and set the pressure cooker mode to "Steam." Cook for 20 minutes. When the cooking time ends, remove the dish from the pressure cooker and place on a serving dish.

Nutritional Information: Calories: 321, Fat: 24.4g, Carbohydrates: 10.9g, Protein: 16g

Almond Muffins

Servings: 6

Preparation Time: 40 minutes

Ingredients:

- 8 Tbsp butter
- ½ cup Baking Stevia
- 1 egg
- 1 tsp vanilla
- 2 cups coconut flour
- 2 tsp baking powder
- 1 tsp salt
- ½ cup chopped almonds
- ½ cup buttermilk

Directions:

1. Use an electric mixer to cream the butter and stevia together until they are light and fluffy.
2. Mix the vanilla and eggs in a small bowl then add to the mixer with the butter blend. Mix until just combined
3. Add the remaining dry ingredients to the mixer and fold together by hand. Add the buttermilk and mix until smooth.
4. Add the almonds to the batter and mix briefly. Pour the muffin batter into eight silicone muffin cups.
5. Place the muffin cups inside the Ninja Foodi on top of a metal trivet. Press the air crisp button and set the temperature to 350 degrees and program the timer to 25 minutes. Once cooked, a toothpick should come out of the center of the cake cleanly. Allow to cool and serve.

Nutritional Information: Calories: 238, Fat: 26g, Carbohydrates: 29g, Protein: 6g

Artichoke Frittata

Servings: 4

Preparation Time: 40 minutes

Ingredients:

- 2 tbsp unsalted butter
- ¼ large yellow bell pepper, chopped
- ½ small red onion, chopped
- 1 cup coarsely chopped artichoke hearts
- 8 large eggs
- Salt and freshly ground black pepper to taste
- ¼ cup almond milk
- ¾ cup shredded Swiss cheese, divided
- ¼ cup grated Parmesan cheese

Directions

1. Select Sear/Sauté mode, adjust to Medium, and choose Start/Stop to preheat the pot for 5 minutes.
2. Melt the butter in the inner pot and sauté the bell pepper, onion, and artichoke hearts until the onion and peppers soften, 5 minutes.
3. Meanwhile, in a medium bowl, whisk the eggs with salt, black pepper, and allow sitting for 1 minute.
4. Whisk in the almond milk and then mix in the half of the Swiss cheese.
5. Pour the egg mixture over the vegetables and stir to evenly distribute the eggs.
6. Allow cooking (undisturbed) until the edges are set, 7 to 9 minutes. Pierce any bubbles that form using the spatula to let out air from the frittata.
7. Press Stop to cancel the Sear/Sauté function and run the spatula in and around the edges of the frittata.
8. Close the Air Crisping Lid; choose Bake/Roast and set the temperature to 375°F, and time to 3 minutes.

9. Press Start to begin baking. After 1 minute, open the lid and sprinkle the remaining Swiss cheese and the Parmesan cheese on the frittata.
10. Close the lid and cook for the remaining 2 minutes. Once the timer ends, carefully open the lid and rest the frittata for 2 minutes. Slice into wedges and serve.

Nutritional Information: Calories: 296, Fat: 21.7g, Carbohydrates: 10.17g, Protein: 15.64g

Stuffed Buns with Egg

Servings: 6

Preparation Time: 18 minutes

Ingredients:

- 3 large keto bread rolls
- 4 eggs
- 7 ounces cheddar cheese
- 1 teaspoon salt
- ½ teaspoon red chili flakes
- ½ teaspoon sour cream
- 1 tablespoon butter

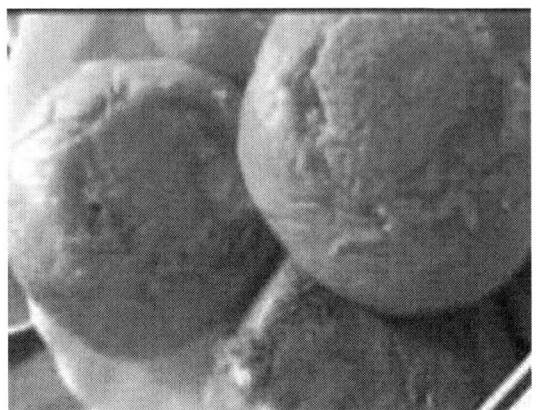

Directions:

1. Cut the keto bread rolls in half. Hollow out the center of the bread half partially. Combine the salt, chili flakes, and sour cream together and stir gently.
2. Add the eggs to a mixing bowl and whisk. Add the butter in the pressure cooker. Pour the eggs equally into the keto bread roll halves.
3. Transfer the bread in the pressure cooker. Sprinkle the dish with the spice mixture. Grate the cheddar cheese and sprinkle the bread with the grated cheese.
4. Close the lid, and set the pressure cooker mode to "Steam." Cook for 10 minutes. Let the dish rest before serving it.

Nutritional Information: Calories: 259, Fats: 19.2g, Carbohydrates: 2.6g, Protein: 17.5g

Bacon, Avocado and Cheese

Servings: 4

Prep Time: 15 minutes

Ingredients:

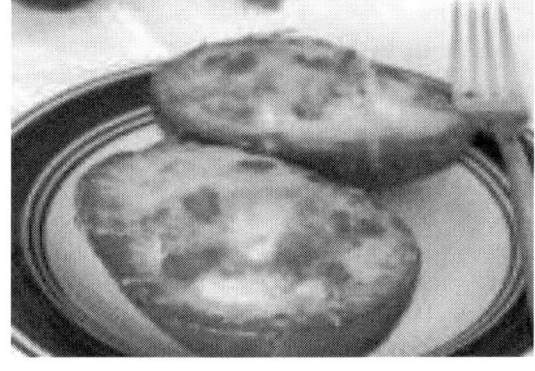

- 8 slices bacon
- 2 Avocados, sliced
- ½ cup cheddar cheese
- ¼ tsp ground black pepper

Directions:

1. Prepare a baking pan that fits in your Ninja Foodi bowl by greasing the pan with butter. Set aside
2. Lay the bacon strips inside the Ninja Foodi, trying not to layer them on top of each other. Set the Ninja Foodi to air crisp at 325 for 7 minutes. Remove the pan of bacon from the Ninja Foodi and place the sliced avocado on top.
3. Sprinkle the top with the cheese and with the ground black pepper. Return to the Foodi and cook for another 2 minutes to melt the cheese. Remove and enjoy while hot!

Nutritional Info: Calories Per Serving: 265, Carbohydrates: 8g, Fats: 23g, Protein: 10g,

Cheesy Hash

Servings: 6

Preparation Time: 35 minutes

Ingredients:

- 6 eggs
- 4 cups riced cauliflower
- ¼ cup milk
- 1 onion, chopped
- 3 Tbsp butter
- 1 ½ cups cheddar cheese

Directions:

1. Press the sauté button on your Ninja Foodi and add the butter and the onions. Cook, stirring occasionally until the onions are soft, about 5 minutes.
2. Add the riced cauliflower to the pot and stir. Turn on the air crisper for 15 minutes, turning the cauliflower halfway through.
3. In a small bowl, mix the eggs and milk together then pour over the browned cauliflower. Sprinkle the cheddar cheese on top and close the lid of the Ninja Foodi for one minute to just melt the cheese. Serve while hot

Nutritional Information (per serving): Calories: 291, Fats: 22g, Carbohydrates: 8g, Protein: 18g

Cheese Casserole

Servings: 2

Preparation Time: 25 minutes

Ingredients

- 1 oz bacon, chopped
- 2 eggs, whisked
- ¼ cup almond milk
- ½ teaspoon dried basil
- 3 oz Cheddar cheese

Directions

1. Mix up together the whisked eggs, almond milk and dried basil.
2. Add bacon and transfer the mixture into the springform pan.
3. Grate cheese and sprinkle it over the egg mixture.
4. Place the casserole into the Foodi and set "Air Crisp "mode 365 F.
5. Cook the casserole for 15 minutes.
6. Check the casserole and cook it for 5-7 minutes more.
7. Serve it!

Nutritional Information: Calories: 380, Fats: 31.5g, Carbohydrates: 2.8g, Protein: 22.1g

Western Omelet

Servings: 2

Preparation Time: 40 minutes

Ingredients

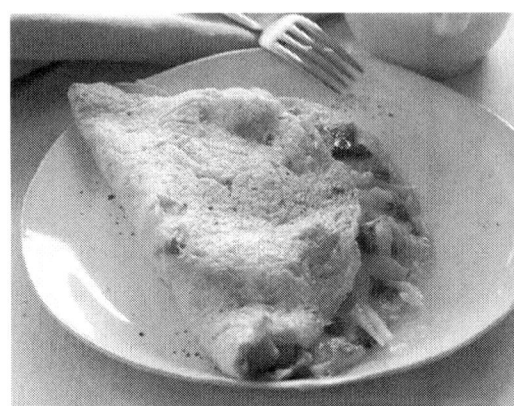

- 3 eggs, whisked
- 5 tablespoon almond milk
- 3 oz chorizo, chopped
- 1 green pepper, chopped ¼ teaspoon salt
- ¾ teaspoon chili flakes
- 1 oz Feta cheese, crumbled

Directions

1. Mix up together all the ingredients and stir gently.
2. Pour the mixture into the omelet pan.
3. Preheat Ninja Foodi at "Roast/Bake" mode at 320 F for 4 minutes.
4. Then transfer the pan with an omelet in Ninja Foodi and cook at the same mode for 30 minutes.
5. Serve the cooked meal hot!

Nutritional Information: Calories: 424, Fat: 34.9g, Carbohydrates: 6.8g, Protein: 21.9g

Creamy Early Morning Asparagus Soup

Servings: 4

Preparation Time: 20 minutes

Ingredients

- 1 tablespoon olive oil
- 3 green onions, sliced crosswise into ¼ inch pieces
- 1-pound asparagus, tough ends removed, cut into 1-inch pieces
- 4 cups vegetable stock
- 1 tablespoon unsalted butter
- 1 tablespoon almond flour
- 2 teaspoon salt
- 1 teaspoon white pepper
- ½ cup heavy cream

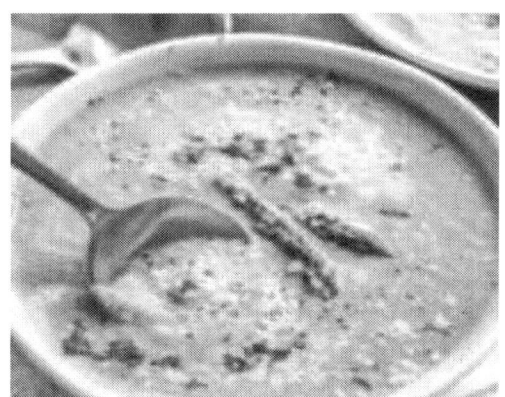

Directions

1. Set your Ninja Foodi to "Sauté" mode and add oil, let it heat up
2. Add green onions and Sauté for a few minutes, add asparagus and stock
3. Lock lid and cook on HIGH pressure for 5 minutes
4. Take a small saucepan and place it over low heat, add butter, flour and stir until the mixture foams and turns into a golden beige, this is your blond roux
5. Remove from heat
6. Release pressure naturally over 10 minutes
7. Open lid and add roux, salt and pepper to the soup
8. Use an immersion blender to puree the soup
9. Taste and season accordingly, swirl in cream and enjoy!

Nutritional Information (per serving): Calories: 192, Fat: 14g, Carbohydrates: 8g, Protein: 6g

Amazing Bacon and Veggie Delight

Servings: 4

Preparation Time: 30 minutes

Ingredients

- 1 green bell pepper, chopped
- 4 bacon slices
- ½ cup parmesan cheese
- 1 tablespoon avocado mayonnaise (Keto Friendly)
- 2 scallions, chopped

Directions

1. Arrange your bacon slices in your Ninja Foodi pot and top them up with avocado mayo, scallions, bell peppers, parmesan cheese
2. Close lid and select the Bake/Roast mode, set timer to 25 minutes and temperature to 365 degrees F
3. Let it bake and remove the dish after 25 minutes
4. Serve and enjoy!

Nutritional Information (Per serving): Calories: 197, Fat: 13g, Carbohydrates: 5g, Protein: 14g

Quiche Lorainde

Servings: 4

Preparation Time: 25 minutes

Ingredients

- 4 eggs, whisked
- ½ teaspoon salt
- ½ teaspoon cayenne pepper
- ¼ cup heavy cream
- 2 oz bacon, chopped
- 1 tablespoon butter
- 3oz Parmesan, grated
- ½ teaspoon dried basil

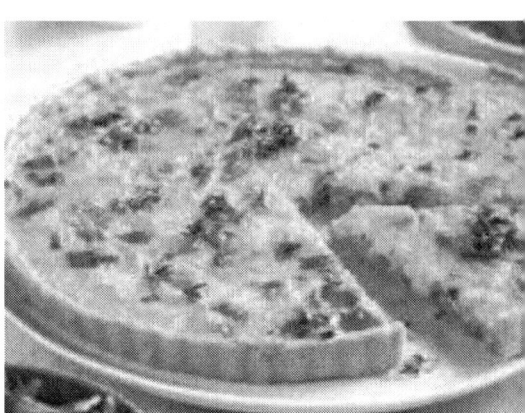

Directions

1. Preheat Ninja Foodi at "Sauté/Stear" mode for 5 minutes.
2. Then add butter and melt it. Add bacon and sauté it for 4 minutes.
3. Meanwhile, whisk together the eggs, salt, cayenne pepper, dried basil, and heavy cream. When the bacon is cooked – add the egg mixture and lower the air fryer lid.
4. Cook the meal for 10 minutes at 365 F.
5. Then top the egg mixture with the grated cheese and cook for 5 minutes more. Serve it!

Nutritional Information: Calories: 260, Fat: 20.5g, Carbohydrates: 1.6g, Protein: 17.8g

Bacon Jalapeno

Servings: 3

Preparation Time: 10 minutes

Ingredients

- 6 jalapeno peppers
- 1 teaspoon minced garlic
- 6 tablespoon cream cheese
- 6 bacon strips, chopped, cooked
- ½ teaspoon salt
- 1 oz ground beef, cooked
- ¼ teaspoon ground cumin

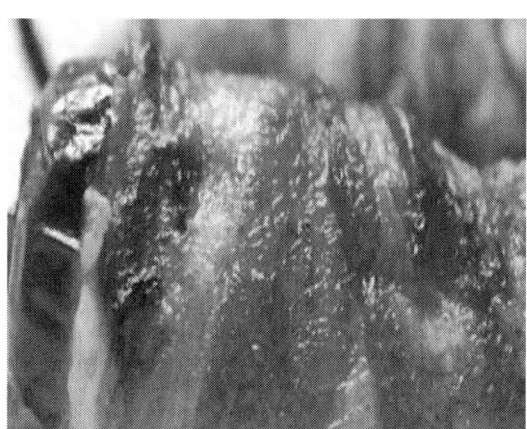

Directions
1. Trim the ends of the peppers and remove all the seeds from inside.
2. Mix up together the minced garlic, cream cheese, salt, and ground cumin. Add the ground beef and stir well. Add bacon.
3. Fill the peppers with the mixture and transfer on the rack.
4. Lower the air fryer lid and cook the jalapenos for minutes at 365 F.
5. Serve the meal immediately!

Nutritional Information: Calories: 301, Fat: 26g, Carbohydrates: 3g, Protein: 12.9g

Egg Caprese Breakfast Cups

Servings: 3

Preparation Time: 10 minutes

Ingredients

- 2 thin slices ham
- 1 tsp dried basil
- 2 tbsp shredded mozzarella cheese
- 2 cherry tomatoes, halved
- Salt and freshly ground black pepper to taste

Directions

1. Line 2 medium ramekins with one ham each, crack in an egg each and top with the basil, mozzarella, and tomatoes.
2. Season with salt, black pepper, and cover with foil; crimp foil.
3. Pour 1 cup of water in inner pot, fix in the reversible rack in the bottom position, and place the ramekins on top.
4. Cover with the Pressure Lid and lock the vent to Seal. Select Pressure, adjust to High and set the timer to 5 minutes.
5. Press Start to cook. After cooking, perform a quick pressure release to let out all the steam and carefully open the lid. Carefully remove the foil.
6. Close the Air Crisping lid and select Bake/Roast. Adjust the temperature to 400°F and the time to 3 minutes.
7. Press Start to brown the top of the eggs.
8. After cooking, open the lid and carefully remove the ramekins. Allow cooling for 3 minutes and serve warm.

Nutritional Information: Calories: 37, Fat: 2.02g, Carbohydrates: 1.54g, Protein: 3.29g

Chapter Five: Chicken and Poultry Recipes

Juicy Sesame Garlic Chicken Wings

Servings: 4

Preparation Time: 35 minutes

Ingredients

- 24 chicken wing segments
- 2 tablespoons toasted sesame oil
- 2 tablespoons Asian-Chile-Garlic sauce
- 2 tablespoons stevia
- 2 garlic cloves, minced
- 1 tablespoon toasted sesame seeds

Directions

1. Add 1 cup water to Foodi's inner pot, place reversible rack in the pot in lower portions, place chicken wings in the rack
2. Place lid into place and seal the valve
3. Select pressure mode to HIGH and cook for 10 minutes
4. Make the glaze by taking a large bowl and whisking in sesame oil, Chile-Garlic sauce, honey and garlic
5. Once the chicken is cooked, quick release the pressure and remove pressure lid
6. Remove rack from the pot and empty remaining water
7. Return inner pot to the base
8. Cover with crisping lid and select Air Crisp mode, adjust the temperature to 375 degrees F, pre-heat for 3 minutes
9. While the Foodi pre-heats, add wings to the sauce and toss well to coat it
10. Transfer wings to the basket, leaving any excess sauce in the bowl

11. Place the basket in Foodi and close with Crisping mode, select Air Crisp mode and let it cook for 8 minutes, gently toss the wings and let it cook for 8 minutes more
12. Once done, drizzle any sauce and sprinkle sesame seeds
13. Enjoy!

Nutritional Information: Calories: 440, Fat: 32g, Carbohydrates: 12g, Protein: 28g

Chicken Salad in Jar

Servings: 10

Preparation Time: 15 minutes

Ingredients

- 1-pound chicken breast, boneless, skinless
- 1 teaspoon ground black pepper
- ½ teaspoon paprika
- ½ teaspoon ground coriander
- 1 tablespoon butter
- 1 cup spinach, chopped
- 1 cucumber, chopped
- 1 teaspoon chili flakes
- 1 teaspoon lemon juice
- 1 teaspoon avocado oil
- 1 cup lettuce, chopped
- 1 cup water for cooking

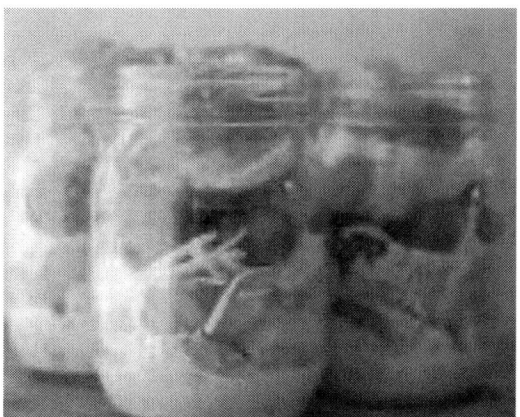

Directions

1. Rub the chicken breast with ground black pepper, paprika, and ground coriander. Then place chicken breast in the cooker.
2. Add water. Close the lid and cook the chicken on High-pressure mode for 15 minutes. Make a quick pressure release.
3. Remove chicken breast from the cooker and chill it little. Meanwhile, in the mixing bowl combine together lettuce and spinach.
4. Sprinkle the greens with chili flakes, lemon juice, and avocado oil.

5. Add cucumber and mix up the mixture. Shred the chicken breast and mix it up with butter. Then fill the serving jars with shredded chicken and add green salad mixture. Store the salad in the fridge.

Nutritional Information: Calories: 174, Fat: 6.1g, Carbohydrates: 4g, Protein: 25g

Tomato Chicken Stew

Preparation time: 50 minutes

Servings: 8

Ingredients

- ½ cup tomato juice
- 1 tablespoon sugar
- 1 teaspoon salt
- 1 pound boneless chicken breast
- 1 tablespoon oregano
- 1 teaspoon cilantro
- 1 teaspoon fresh ginger
- 2 carrots
- 3 red onion
- 5 ounces shallot
- 1 tablespoon ground black pepper
- ½ cup cream
- 3 cups chicken stock
- 3 ounces scallions
- 2 tablespoons olive oil
- 3 ounces eggplants

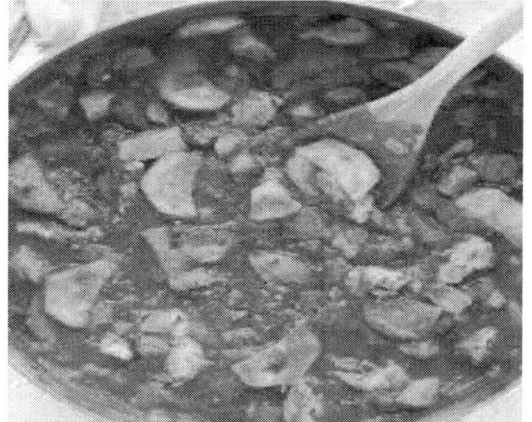

Directions:

1. Combine the tomato juice with the salt, oregano, cilantro, ground black pepper, and cream together in a mixing bowl and stir. Peel the eggplants, onions, and carrots.
2. Chop the vegetables into medium-sized pieces. Set the pressure cooker to "Sauté" mode.
3. Place the chopped vegetables into the pressure cooker and sprinkle them with the olive oil. Sauté the vegetables for 5 minutes.

4. Add the tomato juice mixture and stir. Chop the shallot and scallions. Add the chopped ingredients into the pressure cooker.
5. Chop the boneless chicken breast roughly and add it into the pressure cooker, then add the chicken stock. Stir well using a spoon and close the pressure cooker lid.
6. Cook the dish on "Sauté" mode for 30 minutes.
7. When the stew is cooked, remove it from the pressure cooker and transfer it to serving bowls.

Nutritional Information: calories 205, fat 9g, carbs 13.7g, protein 18.4g

Chicken Puttanesca

Preparation time: 40 minutes

Servings: 8

Ingredients

- 1 ½ pounds chicken thighs
- ½ cup tomato paste
- 2 tablespoons capers
- 1 teaspoon salt
- 1/2 teaspoons black-eyed peas
- 3 garlic cloves
- 3 tablespoons olive oil
- 4 ounces black olives
- 1 tablespoon fresh basil, chopped
- ½ cup of water

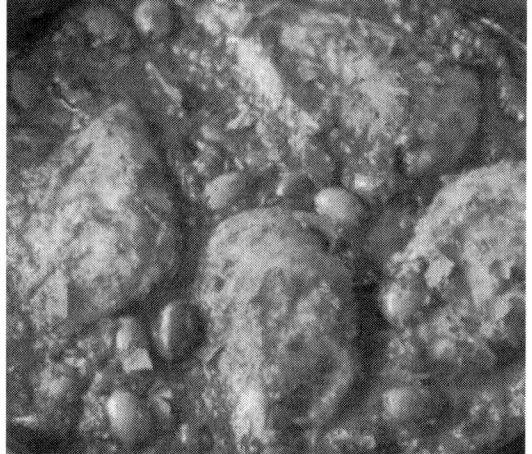

Directions:

1. Set the pressure cooker to "Sauté" mode.
2. Pour the olive oil into the pressure cooker and preheat it for 1 minute. Place the chicken thighs into the pressure cooker and sauté the chicken for 5 minutes. When the chicken thighs are browned, remove them from the pressure cooker.
3. Put the tomato paste, capers, olives, black-eyed peas, and basil into the pressure cooker. Peel the garlic and slice it. Add the sliced garlic to the pressure cooker mixture.
4. Add the salt and water. Stir the mixture well and sauté it for 3 minutes.
5. Add the chicken thighs and close the lid. Cook the dish on "Pressure" mode for 17 minutes. When the cooking time ends, open the pressure cooker lid and transfer the dish to the serving bowl.

Nutritional Information: calories 170, fat 8.8g, carbs 4.48g, protein 18g

Spicy Chicken Strips

Servings: 7

Preparation time: 18 minutes

Ingredients

- 1 cup almond flour
- 1 teaspoon kosher salt
- 1 teaspoon cayenne pepper
- ½ teaspoon cilantro
- ½ teaspoon oregano
- ½ teaspoon paprika
- ½ cup of coconut milk
- 1 pound chicken fillet
- 3 tablespoons sesame oil
- 1 teaspoon turmeric

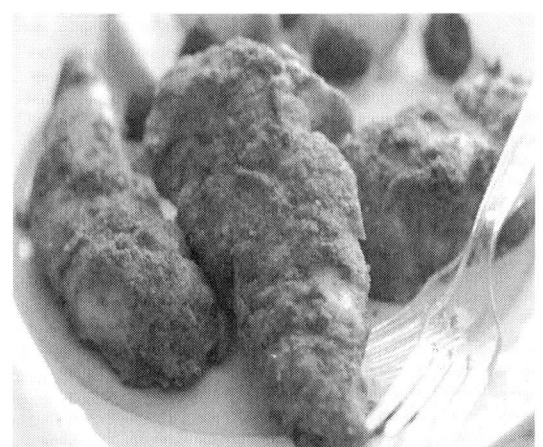

Directions:

1. Place the flour in a mixing bowl. Add kosher salt, cayenne pepper, cilantro, oregano, paprika, and turmeric and mix well. Pour the coconut milk in a separate bowl.
2. Cut the chicken into strips. Set the pressure cooker to "Sauté" mode.
3. Pour the olive oil into the pressure cooker. Dip the chicken strips in the coconut milk, then dip them in the almond flour mixture.
4. Repeat this step two more times.
5. Add the dipped chicken strips to the pressure cooker. Sauté the chicken strips for 3 minutes on each side.
6. Transfer the chicken toa paper towel to drain any excess oil before serving.

Nutritional Information: calories 244, fat 18.1g, carbs 10.6g, protein 11.9g

Chicken and Parsnip

Servings: 4

Preparation time: 45 minutes

Ingredients

- 4 chicken thighs
- Salt to taste
- 2 tsp turmeric powder
- 1 tsp dried oregano
- ½ tsp dry mustard
- 2 tsp Worcestershire sauce
- ¼ tsp sweet paprika
- ¼ tsp hot sauce
- ½ tsp garlic powder
- 2 tbsp melted butter
- ¼ cup chicken stock
- 1 tbsp olive oil
- 1½ lbs medium parsnips, peeled and quartered

Directions

1. Season the chicken on both sides with salt.
2. In a small bowl, combine the turmeric, oregano, mustard, Worcestershire sauce, paprika, hot sauce, garlic powder, butter, and chicken stock. On the Foodi, select Sear/Sauté and adjust to Medium-High. Press Start to preheat the inner pot for 5 minutes.
3. Heat the olive oil in the pot and sear the chicken until golden on the outside, 5 minutes. Transfer to a plate. Stir the parsnips in the chicken fat to be coated well.
4. Put the chicken thighs on top of the parsnips and drizzle with the spice mixture

5. Cover with the Pressure Lid and lock the vent to Seal. Select Pressure; adjust to High and the time to 3 minutes. Press Start to begin cooking.
6. After cooking, perform a quick pressure release, and carefully open the lid. Using tongs, remove the chicken onto the Reversible Rack and scoop out some of the liquid in the inner pot. Stir the parsnips into the remaining sauce and set the rack over.
7. Close the Air Crisping Lid and select Bake/Roast; adjust the temperature to 375°F and the cook time to 16 minutes.
8. Press Start to begin crisping the chicken.
9. When done cooking, open the lid and transfer the parsnips and chicken to a serving platter. Drizzle with some sauce and serve warm.

Nutritional Information: calories 643, fat 41.99g, carbs 25.4g, protein 34.85g

Fragrant Drumsticks

Servings: 7

Preparation time: 22 minutes

Ingredients

- 1 pound chicken drumsticks
- 1 teaspoon salt
- 1 teaspoon paprika
- 1 teaspoon white pepper
- 1 cup of water
- 1 teaspoon thyme ½ teaspoon oregano

Directions:

1. Sprinkle the chicken drumsticks with the salt, paprika, thyme, oregano, and white pepper and stir well. Set the pressure cooker to "Pressure" mode.
2. Place the chicken drumsticks into the pressure cooker and add the water. Close the lid and cook for 18 minutes.
3. When the cooking time ends, release the remaining pressure and open the pressure cooker lid. Remove the drumsticks from the pressure cooker and transfer them to the serving platter.

Nutritional Information: calories 112, fat 3.8g, carbs 0.5gg, protein 17.9g

Chicken Soup

Servings: 8

Preparation Time: 55 minutes

Ingredients

- 2 white onions
- 1 teaspoon salt
- 2 tablespoons sour cream
- 5 cups chicken stock
- ½ cup cream
- 1 teaspoon paprika
- 2 sweet bell pepper
- 1-pound boneless thighs
- 4 carrots

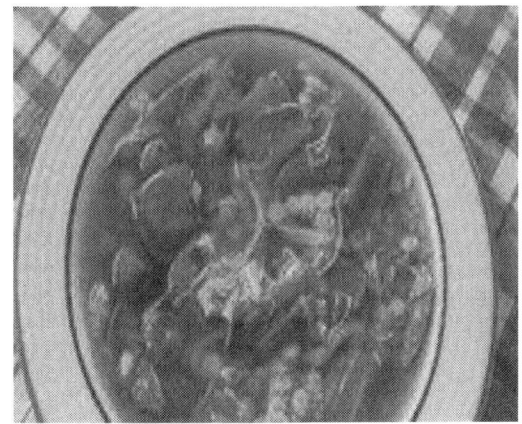

Directions

1. Peel the onion and chop it. Peel the carrot and grate it.
2. Place the cream and chicken stock in the pressure cooker. Add thighs and salt.
3. Close the pressure cooker and cook the mixture on the" Sear/Sauté" mode for 25 minutes.
4. Add the sour cream, chopped onion, and carrot.
5. Remove the seeds from the bell peppers and slice them.
6. Add the sliced peppers in the pressure cooker mixture and close the lid. Cook for 20 minutes.
7. When the soup is cooked, remove it from the pressure cooker and sprinkle the dish with the paprika and serve immediately.

Nutritional Information: Calories: 111, Fat: 3.7g, Carbohydrates: 15.98g, Protein: 6g

Dill Chicken Wings

Serves: 7

Prep time: 30 minutes

Ingredients

- 4 tablespoons dry dill
- 1 cup Greek yogurt
- 1 teaspoon salt
- 1 teaspoon ground black pepper
- ½ teaspoon red chile flakes
- 1 teaspoon oregano
- 1 tablespoon olive oil
- 1 pound chicken wings
- 1 teaspoon lemon juice

Directions:

1. Combine the yogurt, salt, ground black pepper, chili flakes, oregano, and lemon juice together in a mixing bowl, blending until smooth.
2. Add 2 tablespoons of the dill and Stir well. Add the chicken wings and Coat them with the yogurt mixture.
3. Let the chicken wings rest for 2 hours. Set the pressure cooker to «Pressure" mode. Pour the olive oil into the pressure cooker.
4. Add the chicken wings. Sprinkle the chicken wings with the remaining dill. Close the pressure cooker and cook for 20 minutes.
5. When the chicken wings are cooked, remove them from the pressure cooker. Let the wings rest briefly and serve.

Nutritional Information: calories 122, fat 4.5g, carbs 2.77g, protein 17g

Lemon and Butter Chicken Extravagant

Servings: 4

Preparation Time: 20 minutes

Ingredients

- 4 bone-in, skin on chicken thighs
- salt and pepper as needed
- 2 tablespoons butter, divided
- 2 teaspoons garlic, minced
- 1/2 cup herbed chicken stock
- 1/2 cup heavy whip cream
- 1/2 a lemon, juiced

Directions

1. Season chicken thighs with salt and pepper
2. Set your Ninja Foodi to Sauté mode and add oil, let it heat up
3. Add chicken thighs and sauté both sides until golden, total for 6 minutes
4. Remove thighs to a platter and keep it on the side
5. Add garlic and cook for 2 minutes
6. Whisk in chicken stock, heavy cream, lemon juice and stir, bring the sauce to simmer and reintroduce the chicken
7. Lock lid and cook for 10 minutes on HIGH pressure
8. Release pressure naturally over 10 minutes
9. Serve warm and enjoy!

Nutritional Information: Calories: 294, Fat: 26g, Carbohydrates: 4g, Protein: 12g

Salsa Verde Chicken

Servings: 6

Preparational time: 40 minutes

Ingredients

- 10 ounces Salsa Verde
- 1 tablespoon paprika
- 1 pound boneless chicken breasts
- 1 teaspoon salt
- 1 teaspoon ground coriander
- 1 teaspoon cilantro

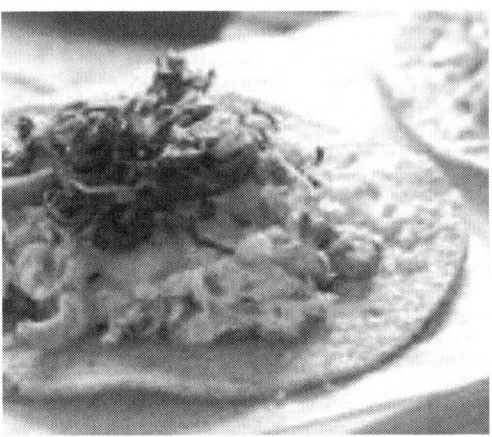

Directions:

1. Rub the boneless chicken breasts with the paprika, salt, ground black pepper, and cilantro. Set the pressure cooker to "Pressure" mode.
2. Place the boneless chicken into the pressure cooker. Sprinkle the meat with the salsa verde and stir well.
3. Close the pressure cooker lid and cook for 30 minutes. When the cooking time ends, release the pressure and transfer the chicken to the mixing bowl. Shred the chicken well. Serve it.

Nutritional Information: calories 222, fat 11.3g, carbs 21.02g, protein 9g

Cheddar Chicken Fillets

Servings: 7

Preparation time: 25 minutes

Ingredients

- 1 cup cream cheese
- 6 ounces Cheddar cheese
- 1 yellow onion
- 14 ounces boneless chicken breast
- 1 teaspoon olive oil
- 1 tablespoon ground black pepper
- 1 teaspoon red chile flakes
- 4 ounces apricot, pitted
- 3 tablespoons chicken stock

Directions:

1. Cut the chicken breast into fillets and sprinkle the boneless chicken breasts with the ground black pepper, olive oil, and chile flakes. Set the pressure cooker to "Sauté" mode.
2. Transfer the chicken breasts into the pressure cooker and sauté the dish for 5 minutes on both sides.
3. Meanwhile, grate the Cheddar cheese and combine it with the cream cheese. Add chicken stock and mix well using a spoon. Peel the onion and slice it.
4. Chop the apricots and combine them with the sliced onion. When the cooking time ends, open the pressure cooker lid. Sprinkle the chicken with the onion mixture.
5. Add the Cheddar cheese mixture. Close the lid and cook the boneless chicken breasts at the "Pressure" mode for 10 minutes.
6. When the cooking time ends, release the remaining pressure and open the pressure cooker lid. Transfer the chicken to the serving plates.

Nutrition: calories 282, fat 18.1g, fiber 1g, carbs 11.88g, protein 18g

Thai Chicken Fillet

Preparation time: 45 minutes

Servings: 8

Ingredients

- 14 ounces boneless chicken breast
- 1 teaspoon ground black pepper
- 1 teaspoon paprika
- 1 teaspoon turmeric
- 3 tablespoons fish sauce
- ½ teaspoon curry
- 1 teaspoon salt
- 3 tablespoons butter
- ¼ cup fresh basil
- 1 teaspoon olive oil

Directions:

1. Cut the boneless chicken breast into medium pieces. Combine the ground black pepper, paprika, turmeric, curry, and salt together in a mixing bowl and stir well.
2. Sprinkle the chicken with the spice mixture and Stir well. Chop the basil and combine it with the butter in a small bowl. Stir the mixture until smooth. Set the pressure cooker to "Sauté" mode.
3. Add the butter mixture into the pressure cooker. Melt it. Transfer the chicken filets into the pressure cooker and sauté them for 10 minutes. Add the olive oil and fish sauce.
4. Close the pressure cooker lid and cook the dish on «Sear/Sauté" mode for 25 minutes. When the dish is cooked, remove the chicken from the pressure cooker.
5. Let the dish rest briefly and serve.

Nutritional Information: calories 182, fat 12g, carbs 12.7g, protein 6g

BBQ Chicken Balls

Servings: 8`

Preparation Time: 45 minutes

Ingredients

- ⅓ cup BBQ sauce
- 1 teaspoon salt
- 1 teaspoon sugar
- 3 tablespoons chives
- 12 ounces ground chicken
- 1 egg
- 1 tablespoon coconut flour
- 1 tablespoon olive oil
- 1 teaspoon oregano
- 1 red onion

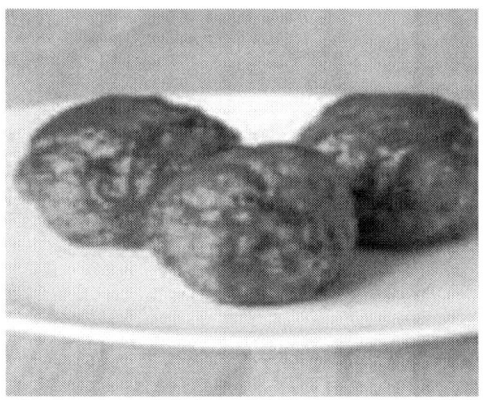

Directions:

1. Put the ground chicken in a mixing bowl. Sprinkle the ground meat with the sugar, salt, chives, coconut flour, and oregano.
2. Peel the red onion, dice it, and add the onion to the ground chicken mixture. Beat the egg and add it to the ground chicken. Mix everything well using your hands until smooth. Make small balls from the ground chicken. Set the pressure cooker to "Sauté" mode.
3. Pour the olive oil into the pressure cooker. Put the chicken balls in the pressure cooker and sauté them for 5 minutes.
4. Stir them constantly to make all the sides of the chicken balls are brown.
5. Pour the barbecue sauce into the pressure cooker and close the lid. Cook the dish on «Sear/Sauté" mode for 20 minutes. When the cooking time ends, remove the dish from the pressure cooker and serve.

Nutritional Information: calories 131, fat 5.7g, carbs 6.3g, protein 13.3g

Stuffed Chicken Caprese

Servings: 6

Preparation Time: 45 minutes

Ingredients

- 13 oz chicken breast, skinless, boneless
- 1 tomato, sliced
- ½ cup fresh basil
- 5 oz Mozzarella, sliced
- ½ teaspoon salt
- 1 tablespoon butter
- 1 teaspoon paprika
- 1 tablespoon olive oil
- 1 teaspoon chili flakes
- ½ teaspoon turmeric
- 1 cup water, for cooking

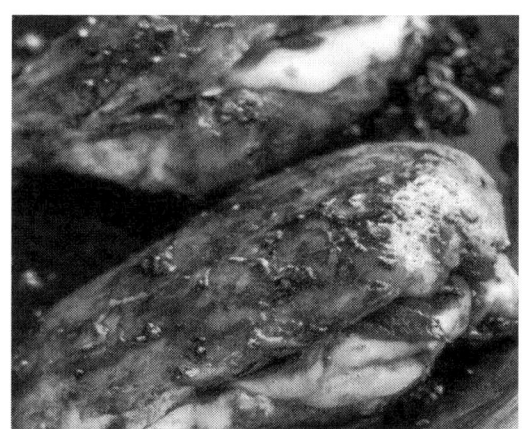

Directions

1. Beat the chicken breast gently with the help of the smooth side of the kitchen hammer. Then make a longitudinal cut in the breast (to get the pocket).
2. Chop the fresh basil roughly. Rub the chicken breast with salt, paprika, chili flakes, and turmeric. Then fill it with sliced Mozzarella, butter, and chopped fresh basil.
3. Brush the chicken breast with olive oil and wrap into the foil. Pour water in the Ninja cooker and insert trivet.
4. Transfer the chicken breast on the trivet and close the lid. Cook the meal on High-pressure mode for 30 minutes.
5. After this, use quick pressure release and discard foil from the chicken. Slice it and transfer on the serving plates.

Nutritional Information: Calories: 182, Fat: 11.2g, Carbohydrates: 1.3g, Protein: 18.5g

Breast with Pomegranate Sauce

Servings: 6

Prep time: 40 minutes

Ingredients

- ½ cup pomegranate juice
- 2 tablespoons Erythritol
- 1 teaspoon cinnamon
- ¼ cup chicken stock
- 2 pounds of chicken breast
- 1 teaspoon starch
- 1 teaspoon butter
- 1 tablespoon oregano
- 1 teaspoon turmeric
- ½ teaspoon red chili flakes

Directions:

1. Set the pressure cooker to "Pressure" mode.
2. Put the chicken breast into the pressure cooker and sprinkle it with the oregano, butter, chicken stock, and chile flakes. Stir the mixture and close the pressure cooker lid. Cook the meat for 20 minutes.
3. Combine the pomegranate juice, Erythritol, cinnamon, starch, and turmeric and stir well until everything is dissolved. When the cooking time ends, open the pressure cooker lid and remove the chicken. Set the pressure cooker to "Sauté" mode. Pour the pomegranate sauce into the pressure cooker and sauté it for 4 minutes, Return the chicken back into the pressure cooker and stir the dish using a spoon.
4. Close the lid and cook the chicken on "Pressure" mode for 5 minutes. When the cooking time ends, release the remaining pressure and open the pressure cooker lid.

5. Transfer the dish to a serving plate and sprinkle it with the pomegranate sauce.

Nutritional Information: calories 198, fat 4.6g, fiber 0.6g, carbs 4.7g, protein 32.2g

Spicy Hot Paprika Chicken

Servings: 4

Preparation Time: 15 minutes

Ingredients

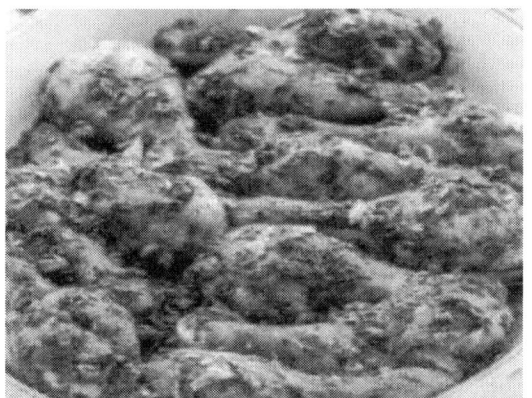

- 4 pieces (4 ounces each) chicken breast, skin on
- Salt and pepper as needed
- 1 tablespoon olive oil
- ½ cup sweet onion, chopped
- ½ cup heavy whip cream
- 2 teaspoons smoked paprika
- ½ cup sour cream
- 2 tablespoons fresh parsley, chopped

Directions

1. Lightly season the chicken with salt and pepper
2. Set your Ninja Foodi to Sauté mode and add oil, let the oil heat up
3. Add chicken and sear both sides until properly browned, should take about 15 minutes
4. Remove chicken and transfer them to a plate
5. Take a skillet and place it over medium heat, add onion and Sauté for 4 minutes until tender
6. Stir in cream, paprika and bring the liquid simmer
7. Return chicken to the skillet and alongside any juices
8. Transfer the whole mixture to your Ninja Foodi and lock lid, cook on HIGH pressure for 5 minutes
9. Release pressure naturally over 10 minutes
10. Stir in sour cream, serve and enjoy!

Nutritional Information: Calories: 389, Fat: 30g, Carbohydrates: 4g, Protein: 25g

Oregano Chicken Wings

Servings: 6

Preparation Time: 25 minutes

Ingredients

- 12 chicken wings, bones removed
- 1 tablespoon oregano
- 1 teaspoon paprika
- 1 teaspoon turmeric
- ½ teaspoon salt
- 2 tablespoons butter, melted
- 1 teaspoon cayenne pepper
- ½ teaspoon olive oil
- ½ teaspoon minced garlic

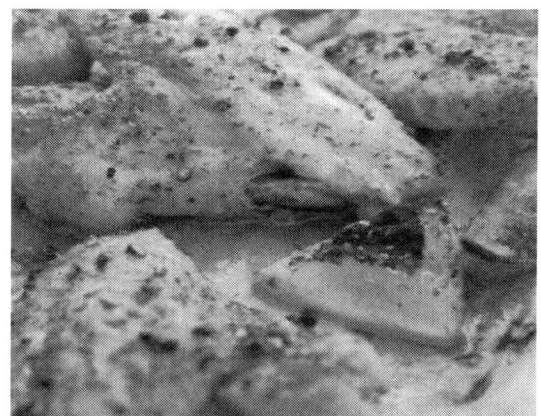

Directions

1. Make the chicken marinade: mix up together oregano, paprika, turmeric, salt, melted butter, cayenne pepper, olive oil, and minced garlic.
2. Whisk the mixture well. Then brush every chicken wing with marinade and leave for 10 minutes to marinate.
3. After this, transfer the chicken wings into the cooker basket and lower the crisp lid. Cook the chicken wings for 10 minutes or until they are light brown.

Nutritional Information: Calories: 361, Fat: 25.8g, Carbohydrates: 11.9, Protein: 19.7g

Chicken Bread

Servings: 8

Preparation time: 45 minutes

Ingredients

- ½ tablespoon garam masala powder
- 8 ounces keto dough
- 1 teaspoon sesame seeds
- 1 egg yolk
- 1 teaspoon ground cilantro
- 1 teaspoon dill
- 10 ounces ground chicken
- ¼ cup fresh parsley
- 1 teaspoon olive oil
- 1 tablespoon ground black pepper
- 1 onion

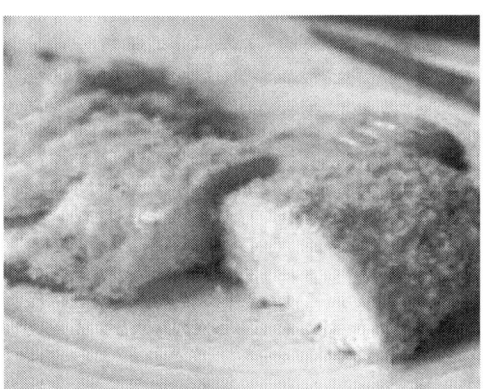

Directions:

1. Roll the dough using a rolling pin. Combine the ground chicken with the ground cilantro and ground black pepper and stir well. Wash the parsley carefully and chop it.
2. Add the parsley to the chicken mixture. Peel the onion and dice it. Add the onion to the chicken mixture.
3. Mix the meat mixture using your hands. Set the pressure cooker to "Pressure" mode. Place the ground meat mixture in the middle of the rolled dough.
4. Wrap the dough in the shape of the bread. Spray the pressure cooker with the olive oil inside and put the chicken bread there.
5. Whisk the egg yolk and sprinkle the chicken bread with it. Sprinkle the dish with the sesame seeds.

6. Close the pressure cooker lid and cook the dish for 40 minutes. When the cooking time ends, open the pressure cooker lid and check to see if the dish is cooked using a toothpick.
7. Transfer the chicken bread to a serving plate and let it rest briefly. Slice it and serve.

Nutritional Information: calories 189, fat 5.3g, fiber 4.2g, carbs 8.1g, protein 27.3g

Crunchy Chicken Skin

Servings: 7

Preparation Time: 20 minutes

Ingredients

- 1 teaspoon red chili flakes
- 1 teaspoon ground black pepper
- 1 teaspoon salt
- 9 ounces of chicken's skin
- 2 tablespoons butter
- 1 teaspoon olive oil
- 1 teaspoon paprika

Directions

1. Combine the ground black pepper, chili flakes, and paprika together.
2. Stir the mixture and combine it with the chicken skin. Let the mixture rest for 5 minutes. Set the pressure cooker to" Sauté" mode.
3. Add the butter in the pressure cooker and melt it.
4. Add the chicken skin and sauté it for 10 minutes, stirring frequently. When the chicken skin gets crunchy, remove it from the pressure cooker.
5. Place the chicken skin on the paper towel and drain. Serve warm.

Nutritional Information: Calories: 133, Fat: 11.5g, Carbohydrates: 0.98g, Protein: 7g

Chicken Nuggets

Servings: 6

Preparation Time: 35 minutes

Ingredients

- 2 cups ground chicken
- ½ cup dill
- 1 egg
- 2 tablespoons pork rinds
- 1 tablespoon heavy cream
- ½ cup almond flour
- 3 tablespoons butter
- 1 tablespoon canola oil
- 1 teaspoon ground black pepper

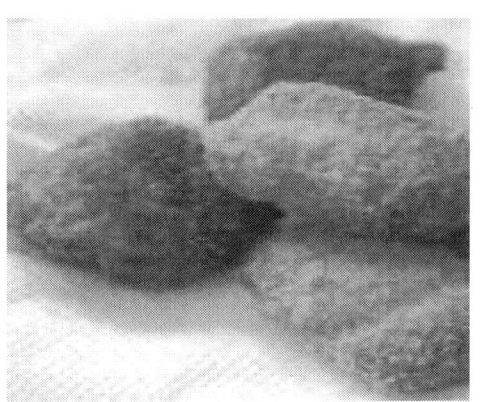

Directions

1. Wash the dill and chop it. Beat the egg in the mixing bowl and whisk it.
2. Add the chopped dill and ground chicken. Blend the mixture until it is smooth.
3. Sprinkle the dish with the ground black pepper and cream. Blend the nugget mixture again. Form the nuggets from the meat mixture and dip them in the almond flour and pork rinds.
4. Sprinkle the pressure cooker with the canola oil and butter.
5. Set the pressure cooker to" Pressure" mode. When the butter mixture starts to melt, add the nuggets.
6. Close the pressure cooker lid and cook the dish for 20 minutes. When the cooking time ends, check if the nuggets are cooked and remove them from the pressure cooker.
7. Drain on paper towel and serve.

Nutritional Information: Calories: 217, Fat: 15.4g, Carbohydrates: 3.1g, Protein: 17.4g

Sour Cream Chicken Liver

Prep time: 18 minutes

Servings: 7

Ingredients

- 1 pound chicken livers
- 1 onion
- 1 teaspoon garlic powder
- 1 tablespoon cilantro
- ¼ cup dill
- 1 teaspoon olive oil
- 1 cup cream
- ¼ cup cream cheese
- 1 teaspoon salt
- 1 teaspoon ground white pepper

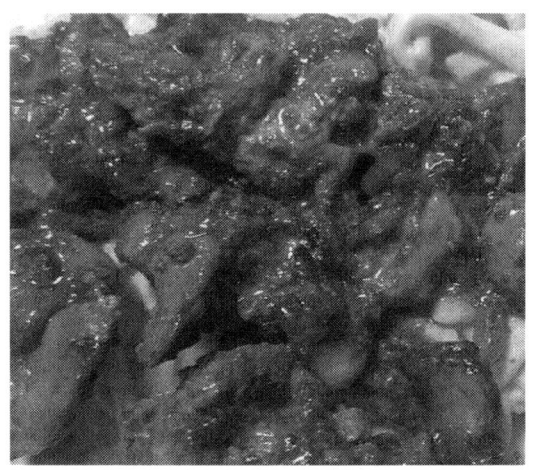

Directions:

1. Chop the chicken livers roughly and place them into the pressure cooker. Set the pressure cooker to "Sauté" mode.
2. Sprinkle the liver with the olive oil and sauté it for 3 minutes, stirring frequently.
3. Combine the sour cream and cream cheese together in a mixing bowl.
4. Sprinkle the mixture with the cilantro, garlic powder, salt, and ground black pepper and stir well. Pour the sour cream mixture into the pressure cooker and stir well.
5. Close the pressure cooker lid and cook the dish on "Sear/Sauté" mode for 15 minutes. When the dish is cooked, let it rest briefly and serve.

Nutritional Information: calories 239, fat 18.2, carbs 8.22, protein 11

Ham-Stuffed Generous Turkey Rolls

Servings: 8

Preparation Time: 30 minutes

Ingredients

- 4 tablespoons fresh sage leaves
- 8 ham slices
- 8 (6 ounces each) turkey cutlets
- Salt and pepper to taste
- 2 tablespoons butter, melted

Directions

1. Season turkey cutlets with salt and pepper
2. Roll turkey cutlets and wrap each of them with ham slices tightly
3. Coat each roll with butter and gently place sage leaves evenly over each cutlet
4. Transfer them to your Ninja Foodi
5. Lock lid and select the "Bake/Roast" mode, bake for 10 minutes a 360 degrees F
6. Open the lid and gently give it a flip, lock lid again and bake for 10 minutes more
7. Once done, serve and enjoy!

Nutritional Information: Calories: 467, Fat: 24g, Carbohydrates: 1.7g, Protein: 56g

Shredded Chicken in Lettuce

Servings: 6

Preparation Time: 40 minutes

Ingredients

- 8 ounces chicken fillet
- ¼ cup tomato juice
- 5 tablespoon sour cream
- 1 teaspoon ground black pepper
- 8 ounces lettuce leaves
- 1 teaspoon salt
- ½ cup chicken stock
- 1 teaspoon butter
- 1 teaspoon turmeric

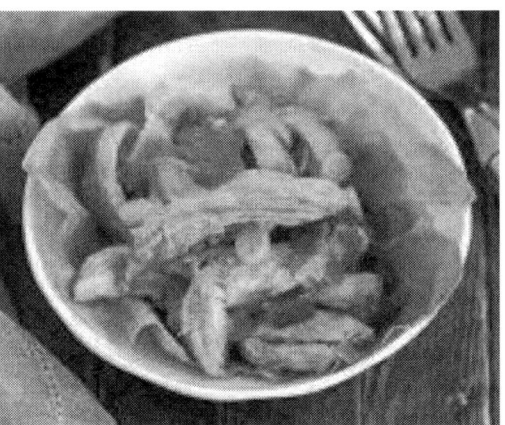

Directions

1. Chop the chicken fillet roughly and sprinkle it with the sour cream, tomato juice, ground black pepper, turmeric, and salt. Mix up the meat mixture.
2. Put the chicken spice mixture in the pressure cooker and add chicken stock.
3. Close the lid and cook the dish on the" Sear/Sauté" mode for 30 minutes. When the chicken is cooked, remove it from the pressure cooker and shred it well.
4. Add the butter and blend well. Transfer the shredded chicken in the lettuce leaves.
5. Serve the dish warm.

Nutritional Information: Calories: 138, Fat: 7.4g, Carbohydrates: 12.63g, Protein: 6g

Sensational Lime and Chicken Chili

Servings: 6

Preparation Time: 23 minutes

Ingredients

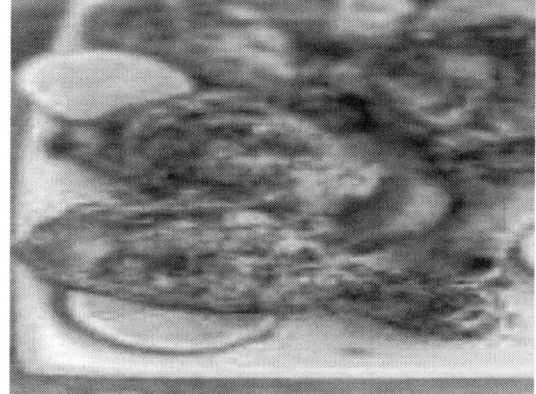

- ¼ cup cooking wine (Keto-Friendly)
- ½ cup organic chicken broth
- 1 onion, diced
- 1 teaspoon salt
- ½ teaspoon paprika
- 5 garlic cloves, minced
- 1 tablespoon lime juice
- ¼ cup butter
- 2 pounds chicken thighs
- 1 teaspoon dried parsley
- 3 green chilies, chopped

Directions

1. Set your Ninja-Foodi to Sauté mode and add onion and garlic
2. Sauté for 3 minutes, add remaining ingredients
3. Lock lid and cook on Medium-HIGH pressure for 20 minutes
4. Release pressure naturally over 10 minutes
5. Serve and enjoy!

Nutritional Information: Calories: 282, Fat: 15g, Carbohydrates: 6g, Protein: 27g

Aromatic Whole Chicken

Servings: 9

Preparation Time: 45 minutes

Ingredients

- 2 pounds whole chicken
- 1 tablespoon salt
- 1 teaspoon ground black pepper
- 1 tablespoon olive oil
- 1 teaspoon butter
- 1 teaspoon fresh rosemary
- 1 lemon
- 1 tablespoon sugar
- 1 cup of water
- 1 teaspoon coriander
- ½ teaspoon cayenne pepper
- ¼ teaspoon turmeric

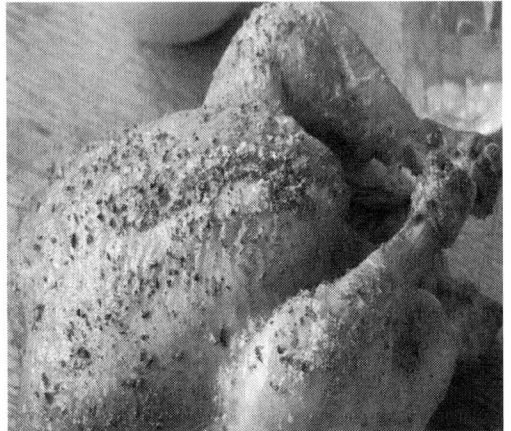

Directions

1. Wash the chicken thoroughly, removing the neck and gizzards if still inside the cavity.
2. Combine the salt, ground black pepper, fresh rosemary, sugar, coriander, cayenne pepper, and turmeric together in a mixing bowl and stir.
3. Rub the chicken with the spice mixture. Wash the red apples and chop them, removing the cores.

4. Combine the chopped apples with the butter and stuff the chicken with the fruit mixture. Sprinkle the chicken with the olive oil. Set the pressure cooker to" Pressure" mode.
5. Pour the water into the pressure cooker and place the stuffed whole chicken. Close the lid and cook for 30 minutes. When the cooking time ends, release the remaining pressure and open the pressure cooker lid.
6. Remove the chicken from the pressure cooker and let it rest. Cut the chicken into pieces and serve.

Nutritional Information: Calories: 217, Fat: 9.5g, Carbohydrates: 2.3g, Protein: 29.3g

Funky-Garlic And turkey Breasts

Servings: 4

Preparation Time: 27 minutes

Ingredients

- ½ teaspoon garlic powder
- 4 tablespoons butter
- ¼ teaspoon dried oregano
- 1-pound turkey breasts, boneless
- 1 teaspoon pepper
- ½ teaspoon salt
- ¼ teaspoon dried basil

Directions

1. Season turkey on both sides generously with garlic, dried oregano, dried basil, salt and pepper
2. Set your Ninja Foodi to sauté mode and add butter, let the butter melt
3. Add turkey breasts and sauté for 2 minutes on each side
4. Lock the lid and select the "Bake/Roast" setting, bake for 15 minutes at 355 degrees F
5. Serve and enjoy

Nutritional Information: Calories: 223, Fat: 13g, Carbohydrates: 5g, Protein: 19g

Chicken Jerky

Servings: 6

Preparation Time: 12 minutes

Ingredients

- ½ cup coconut aminos
- ½ pound chicken breast, sliced into 1/8" thick strips
- 2 Tbsp. Worcestershire sauce
- 2 tsp. ground black pepper
- 1 tsp. liquid smoke
- 1 tsp. onion powders
- 1 tsp. kosher salt
- ½ tsp. garlic powder

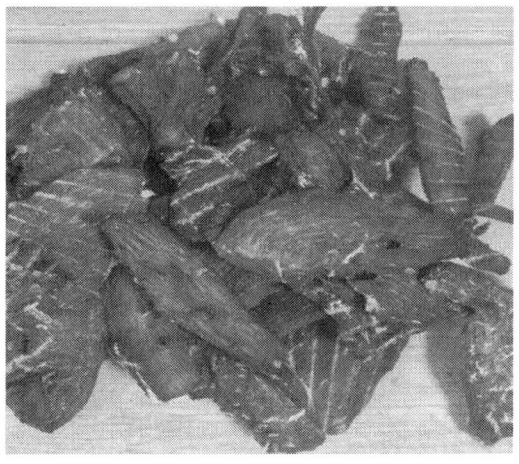

Directions

1. Place all the ingredients in a large Ziploc bag and seal shut. Shake to mix and leave in the fridge overnight.
2. Lay the strips on the dehydrator trays, being careful not to overlap them
3. Place the cook and crisp lid on and set the temperature for 135 degrees for 7 hours. Once done, store in an airtight container.

Nutritional Information: Calories: 67, Fat: 9g, Carbohydrates: 1g, Protein: 4g

Sweet and Sour Chicken Wings

Servings: 4

Preparation Time: 40 minutes

Ingredients

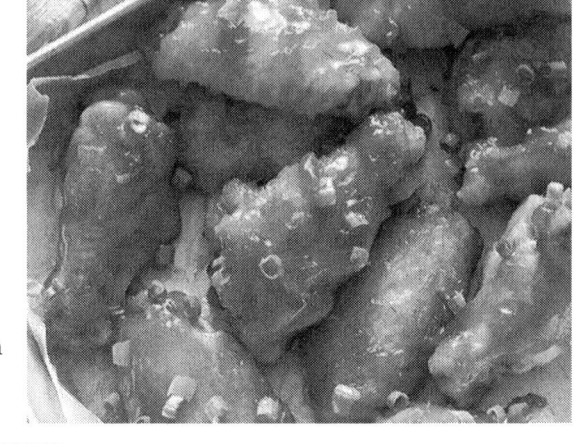

- ½ cup water
- 2 tbsp baking stevia
- 2 tbsp butter
- 2 tbsp lemon juice
- 32 ounces frozen chicken wings
- ½ tsp ground black pepper
- ½ tsp salt

Directions

1. Add all the ingredients into the cook and crisp basket and place the basket inside the Ninja Foodi.
2. Place the pressure cooker lid on top of the pot and close the pressure valve to the seal position. Set the pressure cooker function to high heat and set the timer for 5 minutes
3. Once the cooking cycle is complete, release the pressure quickly by carefully opening the steamer valve
4. Serve hot

Nutritional Information: Calories: 312, Fat: 23g, Carbohydrates: 2g, Protein: 24g

Steamed Chicken Cutlets

Servings: 8

Preparation Time: 35 minutes

Ingredients

- 14 ounces ground chicken
- 1 teaspoon ground black pepper
- 1 teaspoon paprika
- 1 teaspoon cilantro
- 1 teaspoon oregano
- ½ teaspoon minced garlic
- 2 tablespoons starch
- 1 teaspoon red Chile flake
- 1 tablespoon oatmeal flour
- 1 egg

Directions

1. Place the ground chicken in the mixing bowl.
2. Sprinkle it with the ground black pepper, cilantro, and oregano.
3. Add paprika and minced garlic and combine using your hands.
4. Beat the egg in a separate bowl. Add the starch and oatmeal flour to the egg and stir well until smooth. Add the egg mixture to the ground meat.
5. Add the chili flakes and Mix well. Make the medium cutlets from the ground chicken mixture. Set the pressure cooker to" Steam" mode.
6. Transfer the chicken cutlets to the pressure cooker trivet and place the trivet into the pressure cooker.
7. Close the lid and cook the dish on steam mode for 25 minutes. When the dish is cooked, remove the food from the pressure cooker, let it rest, and serve.

Nutritional Information: Calories: 96, Fat: 23g, Carbohydrates: 2g, Protein: 24g

Chapter Six: Keto Ninja Foodi Appetizers and Deserts

Glazed Walnuts

Servings: 4

Preparation time: 10 minutes

Ingredients

- ⅓ cup of water
- 6 ounces walnuts
- 5 tablespoon Erythritol
- ½ teaspoon ground ginger
- 3 tablespoons psyllium husk powder

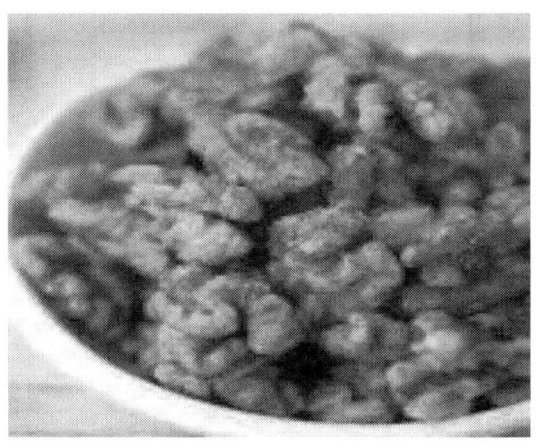

Directions:

1. Combine Erythritol and water together in a mixing bowl. Add ground ginger and stir the mixture until the sugar is dissolved.
2. Transfer the walnuts in the pressure cooker and add sweet liquid. Close the pressure cooker lid and cook the dish on the "Pressure" mode for 4 minutes.
3. Remove the walnuts from the pressure cooker. Dip the walnuts in the Psyllium husk powder and serve.

Nutritional Information: calories 286, fat 25.1g, carbs 10.4g, protein 10.3g

Blackberry Cake

Servings: 4

Preparation Time: 35 minutes

Ingredients

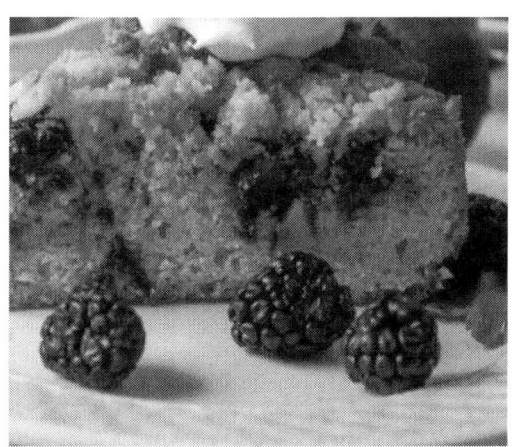

- 4 tablespoons butter
- 3 tablespoon Erythritol
- 2 eggs, whisked
- ½ teaspoon vanilla extract
- 1 oz blackberries
- 1 cup almond flour
- ½ teaspoon baking powder

Directions

1. Combine together all the liquid ingredients.
2. Then add baking powder, almond flour, and Erythritol.
3. Stir the mixture until smooth.
4. Add blackberries and stir the batter gently with the help of the spoon.
5. Take the non-sticky springform pan and transfer the batter inside.
6. Place the springform pan in the pot and lower the air fryer lid.
7. Cook the cake for 20 minutes at 365 F.
8. When the time is over – check the doneness of the cake with the help of the toothpick and cook for 5 minutes more if needed.
9. Chill it little and serve!

Nutritional Information: Calories: 173, Fat: 16.7g, Carbohydrates: 2.2g, Protein: 4.2g

Avocado Mousse

Servings: 7

Preparation Time: 12 minutes

Ingredients

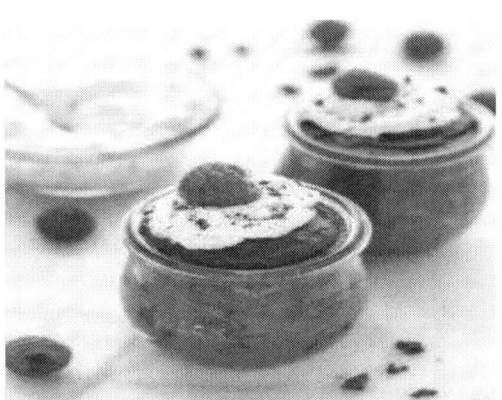

- 2 avocados, peeled, cored
- 1/3 cup heavy cream
- 1 teaspoon of cocoa powder
- 1 teaspoon butter
- 1 teaspoon vanilla extract
- 3 tablespoons Erythritol

Directions

1. Preheat Nin ja Foodi at "Sauté/Stear" mode for 5 minutes.
2. Meanwhile, mash the avocado until smooth and mix it up with Erythritol.
3. Place the butter in the pot and melt.
4. Add mashed avocado mixture and stir well
5. Add cocoa powder and stir until homogenous/ Sauté the mixture for about 3 minutes
6. Meanwhile, whisk the heavy cream on high for 2 minutes.
7. Transfer the cooked avocado mash in the bowl and chill in ice water
8. When the avocado mash reaches room temperature- add whisked heavy cream and vanilla extract. Stir gently to get white-chocolate swirls
9. Transfer the mousse into small cups and chill for 4 hours in the fridge.
10. Serve!

Nutritional Information: Calories: 144, Fat: 13.9g, Carbohydrates: 10.5g, Protein: 1.3g

Cheesy Bombs

Servings: 8

Preparation Time: 20 minutes

Ingredients

- 6 ounces puff pastry
- 1 teaspoon salt
- 8 ounces mozzarella pearls
- 1 egg
- ½ cup coconut flour
- ¼ cup of coconut milk
- ½ teaspoon oregano
- 2 tablespoons butter

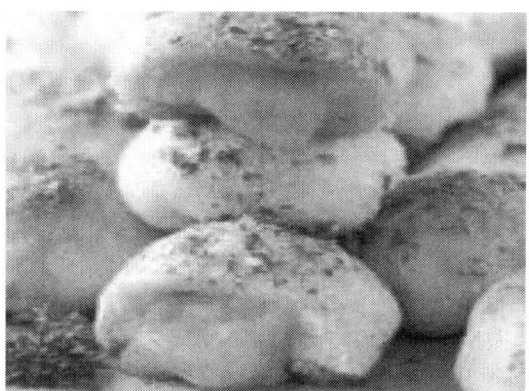

Directions:

1. Roll the puff pastry using a rolling pin. Add the egg to a mixing bowl and blend it using a whisk.
2. Add coconut milk and salt and whisk the mixture until the salt is dissolved. Cut the rolled puff pastry into medium-sized squares.
3. Put a mozzarella pearl in the middle of every square and wrap the dough around each one to make the balls. Sprinkle the egg mixture with the oregano and mix well.
4. Dip the puff pastry balls into the egg mixture, then dip the balls into the coconut flour. Add the butter in the pressure cooker and melt it.
5. Place the puff pastry balls in the pressure cooker and close the lid. Cook the dish on the "Pressure" mode for 10 minutes. When the cooking time ends, release the pressure and open the pressure cooker lid. Transfer the dish to serving plates.

Nutritional Information: Calories: 269, Fat: 19.4g, Carbohydrates: 14.1g, Protein: 8.5g

Cashew Cream

Serves: 10

Preparation time: 18 minutes

Ingredients

- 3 cups cashew
- 2 cups chicken stock
- 1 teaspoon salt
- 1 tablespoon butter
- 2 tablespoons ricotta cheese

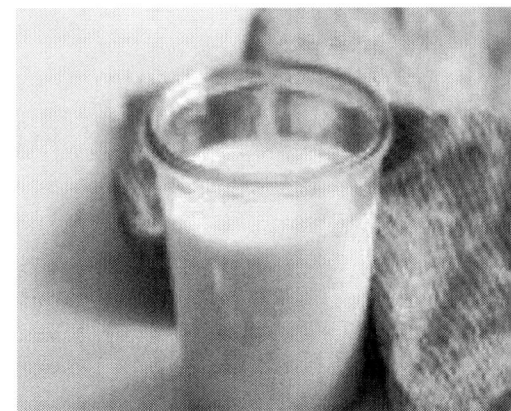

Directions:

1. Combine the cashews with the chicken stock in the pressure cooker.
2. Add salt and close the pressure cooker lid. Cook the dish on the "Pressure" mode for 10 minutes.
3. Remove the cashews from the pressure cooker and drain the nuts from the water. Transfer the cashews to a blender, and add the ricotta cheese and butter.
4. Blend the mixture until it is smooth. When you get the texture you want, remove it from a blender. Serve it immediately or keep the cashew butter in the refrigerator.

Nutritional Information: calories 252, fat 20.6g, carbs 13.8g, protein 6.8g

Broccoli Tots

Servings: 8

Preparation Time: 22 minutes

Ingredients

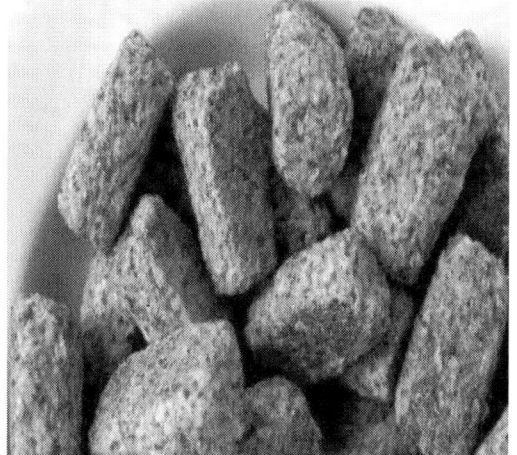

- 1 pound broccoli
- 3 cups of water
- 1 teaspoon salt
- 1 egg
- 1 cup pork rind
- ½ teaspoon paprika
- 1 tablespoon turmeric
- ⅓ cup almond flour
- 2 tablespoons olive oil

Directions:

1. Wash the broccoli and chop it roughly.
2. Put the broccoli in the pressure cooker and add water. Set the pressure cooker to "Steam" mode and steam the broccoli for 20 minutes.
3. Remove the broccoli from the pressure cooker and let it cool. Transfer the broccoli to a blender.
4. Add egg, salt, paprika, turmeric, and almond flour. Blend the mixture until smooth. Add pork rind and blend the broccoli mixture for 1 minute more.
5. Pour the olive oil in the pressure cooker. Form the medium tots from the broccoli mixture and transfer them to the pressure cooker.
6. Set the pressure cooker to "Sauté" mode and cook for 4 minutes on each side. When the dish is cooked, remove the broccoli tots from the pressure cooker and allow them to rest before serving.

Nutritional Information: Calories: 147, Fat: 9.9g, Carbohydrates: 4.7g, Protein: 11.6g

Meatloaf

Serves: 9

Preparation time: 50 minutes

Ingredients

- 2 cups ground beef
- 1 cup ground chicken
- 2 eggs
- 1 tablespoon salt
- 1 teaspoon ground black pepper
- ½ teaspoon paprika
- 1 tablespoon butter
- 1 teaspoon cilantro
- 1 tablespoon basil
- ¼ cup fresh dill

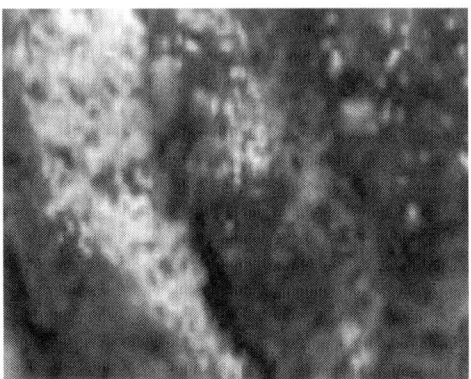

Directions:

1. Combine the ground chicken and ground beef together in a mixing bowl. Add egg, salt, ground black pepper, paprika, butter, and cilantro. Add the basil.
2. Chop the dill and add it to the ground meat mixture and stir using your hands.
3. Place the meat mixture on aluminum foil, shape into a loaf and wrap it. Place it in the pressure cooker. Close the pressure cooker lid and cook the dish on the "Sauté" mode for 40 minutes.
4. When the cooking time ends, remove the meatloaf from the pressure cooker and let it rest. Remove from the foil, slice it, and serve.

Nutritional Information: calories 173, fat 11.5g, carbs 0.81g, protein 16g

Garlic Tomato Slices

Servings: 5

Preparation Time: 15 minutes

Ingredients

- 5 tomatoes
- ¼ cup chives
- ⅓ cup garlic clove
- ½ teaspoon salt
- ½ teaspoon ground black pepper
- 1 tablespoon olive oil
- 7 ounces Parmesan cheese

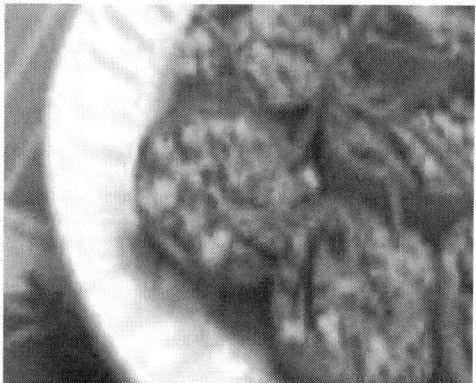

Directions:

1. Wash the tomatoes and slice them into thick slices. Place the sliced tomatoes in the pressure cooker. Chop the chives and grate the Parmesan cheese.
2. Peel the garlic cloves and mince them. Combine the grated cheese and minced garlic and stir the mixture. Sprinkle the tomato slices with the chives, ground black pepper, and salt.
3. Then sprinkle the sliced tomatoes with the cheese mixture. Close the lid and cook the dish on the "Pressure" mode for 5 minutes.
4. When the cooking time ends, remove the tomatoes carefully and serve.

Nutritional Information: Calories: 224, Fat: 14g, Carbohydrates: 12.55g, Protein: 13g

Coconut Pie

Servings: 4

Preparation Time: 16 minutes

Ingredients

- 1 tablespoon coconut flour
- 5 oz coconut, shredded
- ½ teaspoon vanilla extract
- 1 tablespoon Truvia
- 1 teaspoon butter
- 1 egg, whisked
- ¼ cup heavy cream

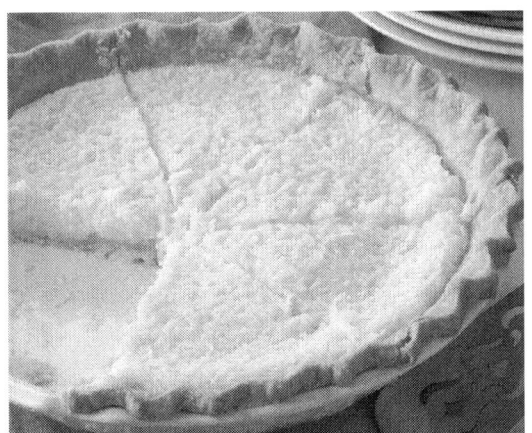

Directions

1. Mix up together the coconut flour, coconut shred, and butter.
2. Stir the mixture until homogenous.
3. Add whisked egg, vanilla extract, Truvia, and heavy cream. Stir well.
4. Transfer the pie mixture into the basket and lower the air fryer lid. Set the Bake mode 355F. Cook the pie for 10 minutes.
5. Check if the pie is cooked with the help of the toothpick and chill it till the room temperature.
6. Serve it!

Nutritional Information: Calories: 185, Fat: 16.9g, Carbohydrates: 8.2g, Protein: 3g

Wrapped Halloumi Cheese

Servings: 8

Preparation Time: 20 minutes

Ingredients

- 1-pound halloumi cheese
- 8 oz bacon, sliced
- 1 teaspoon olive oil

Directions:

1. Cut the cheese into 8 sticks. Wrap every cheese stick into the sliced bacon and sprinkle with olive oil.
2. Place the wrapped sticks in the cooker basket and lower the air fryer lid.
3. Cook the snack for 4 minutes from each side. Serve it warm.

Nutritional Information: Calories: 185, Fat: 16.9g, Carbohydrates: 8.2g, Protein: 3g

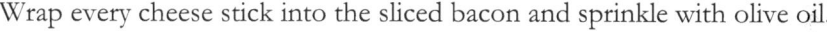

Lava Cups

Servings: 2

Preparation Time: 15 minutes

Ingredients

- 2 eggs, whisked
- 3 tablespoons flax meal
- 2 teaspoons of cocoa powder
- ½ teaspoon baking powder
- 2 tablespoons heavy cream
- Cooking spray

Directions

1. Spray the cake cups with the cooking spray inside.
2. Mix up together all the remaining ingredients and pour the mixture into the prepared cups.
3. Cover the cups with foil and place in Ninja Foodi.
4. Set the Bake mode 355 F.
5. Close the lid and cook the dessert for 8 minutes.
6. Serve the cooked lava cups hot!

Nutritional Information: Calories: 165, Fat: 13.9g, Carbohydrates: 5.3g, Protein: 8.4g

Peanut Butter Cookies

Servings: 7

Preparation Time: 20 minutes

Ingredients

- 1 tablespoon Truvia
- 1 egg, whisked
- 6 oz cashew butter

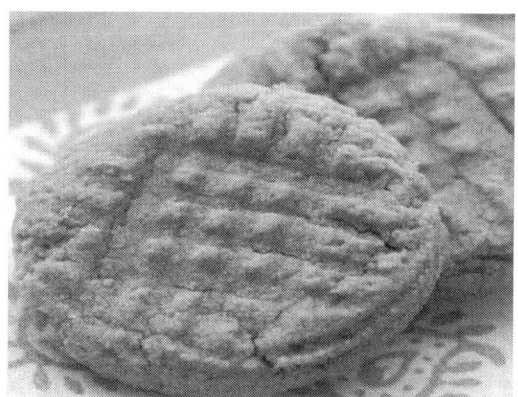

Directions

1. Mix up together all the ingredients and make the small balls.
2. Place the balls in the basket of Ninja Foodi and close the lid.
3. Set the Bake mode and cook the cookies at 330 F for 11 minutes.
4. Increase the time of cooking if you like crunchy cookies. Serve!

Nutritional Information: Calories: 152, Fat: 12.6g, Carbohydrates: 7.4g, Protein: 5.1g

Spinach Dip

Serves: 8

Preparation time: 25 minutes

Ingredients

- 1 cup spinach
- ½ cup cream cheese
- ½ cup cream
- 6 ounces Romano cheese
- 1 teaspoon salt
- 1 teaspoon paprika
- 1 bell pepper
- 1 white medium onion
- 5 tablespoon walnuts
- 1 teaspoon ground ginger
- ½ cup fresh dill

Directions:

1. Wash the spinach and dill and chop the greens. Place the greens in a pressure cooker. Add cream and cream cheese.
2. Grate the Romano cheese and sprinkle the green mixture with the grated cheese. Add the salt, paprika, walnuts, and ground ginger.
3. Remove the seeds from the bell pepper and peel the onion. Chop the vegetables into the same pieces.
4. Add the chopped vegetables in the pressure cooker mixture. Mix up the spinach dip using a spoon carefully. Close the lid and cook the dish on the "Steam" mode for 15 minutes.
5. When the cooking time ends, remove the spinach dip from the pressure cooker and stir until smooth.
6. Place the spinach dip in a serving bowl.

Nutritional Information: calories 196, fat 15.9g, carbs 4.62g, protein 10g

Cauliflower Fritters

Servings: 7

Preparation Time: 28 minutes

Ingredients

- 1 pound cauliflower
- 1 medium white onion
- 1 teaspoon salt
- ½ teaspoon ground white pepper
- 1 tablespoon sour cream
- 1 teaspoon turmeric
- ½ cup dill
- 1 teaspoon thyme
- 3 tablespoons almond flour
- 1 egg
- 2 tablespoons butter

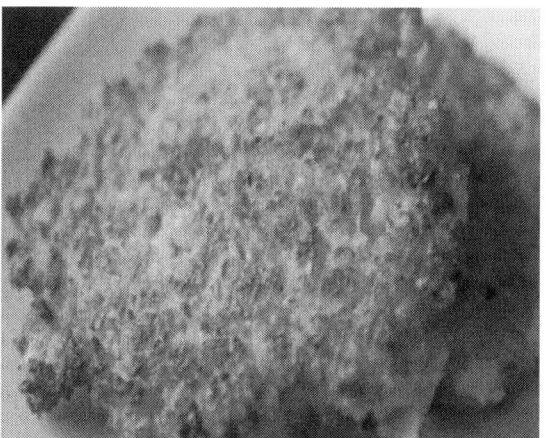

Directions:

1. Wash the cauliflower and separate it into the florets. Chop the florets and place them in a blender. Peel the onion and dice it.
2. Add the diced onion in a blender and blend the mixture. When you get the smooth texture, add salt, ground white pepper, sour cream, turmeric, dill, thyme, and almond flour.
3. Add egg blend the mixture well until a smooth dough forms. Remove the cauliflower dough from a blender and form the medium balls. Flatten the balls a little. Set the pressure cooker to "Sauté" mode.
4. Add the butter in the pressure cooker and melt it. Add the cauliflower fritters in the pressure cooker, and sauté them for 6 minutes. Flip them once.

5. Cook the dish on "Sauté" stew mode for 7 minutes. When the cooking time ends, remove the fritters from the pressure cooker and serve immediately.

Nutritional Information: Calories: 143, Fat: 10.6g, Carbohydrates: 9.9g, Protein: 5.6g

Keto Brownie Batter

Servings: 5

Preparation Time: 15 minutes

Ingredients

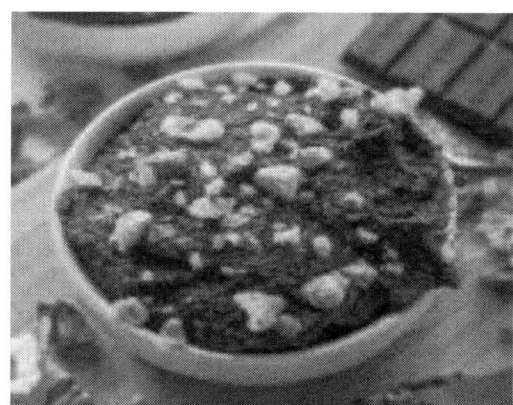

- 1/3 cup almond flour
- 1 tablespoon Erythritol
- ¼ cup heavy cream
- ½ teaspoon vanilla extract
- 3 tablespoons cocoa powder
- 3 tablespoons butter
- 1 oz dark chocolate

Directions

1. Place the almond flour in the springform pan and flatten to make the layer.
2. Then place the springform pan in the pot and lower the air fryer lid.
3. Cook the almond flour for 3 minutes at 400 F or until the almond flour gets a golden color.
4. Meanwhile, combine together cocoa powder and heavy cream; whisk the heavy cream until smooth.
5. Add vanilla extract and Erythritol.
6. Remove the almond flour from Ninja Foodi and chill well.
7. Toss butter and dark chocolate in the pot and preheat for 1 minute on Sauté/Stear mode.
8. When the butter is soft – add it in the heavy cream mixture.
9. Then add chocolate and almond flour.
10. Stir the mass until homogenous and serve!

Nutritional Information: Calories: 159, Fat: 14.9g, Carbohydrates: 9g, Protein: 2.5g

Breadsticks

Servings: 8

Preparation Time: 35 minutes

Ingredients

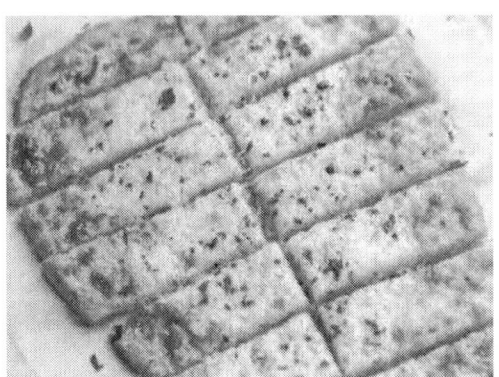

- 1 teaspoon baking powder
- ½ teaspoon Erythritol
- ½ teaspoon salt
- 1 cup of warm water
- 2 cups almond flour
- 5 ounces Parmesan
- 1 tablespoon olive oil
- 1 teaspoon onion powder
- 1 teaspoon basil

Directions:

1. Combine the baking powder, Erythritol, and warm water in a mixing bowl. Stir the mixture well.
2. Add the almond flour, onion powder, salt, and basil. Knead the dough until smooth. Separate dough into 10 pieces and make the long logs. Twist the logs in braids. Grate the Parmesan cheese.
3. Place the twisted logs in the pressure cooker. Sprinkle them with the grated Parmesan cheese and olive oil, and close the lid. Cook the breadsticks at the "Pressure" mode for 10 minutes.
4. When the cooking time ends, release the pressure and open the pressure cooker. Leave the breadsticks for 10 minutes to rest. Serve the breadsticks immediately or keep them in a sealed container.

Nutritional Information: Calories: 242, Fat: 18.9g, Carbohydrates: 2.7g, Protein: 11.7g

Almond Bites

Servings: 5

Preparation Time: 15 minutes

Ingredients

- 1 egg, whisked
- 1 cup almond flour
- ¼ cup almond milk
- 1 tablespoon coconut flakes
- ½ teaspoon vanilla extract
- ½ teaspoon baking powder
- ½ teaspoon apple cider vinegar
- 2 tablespoons butter

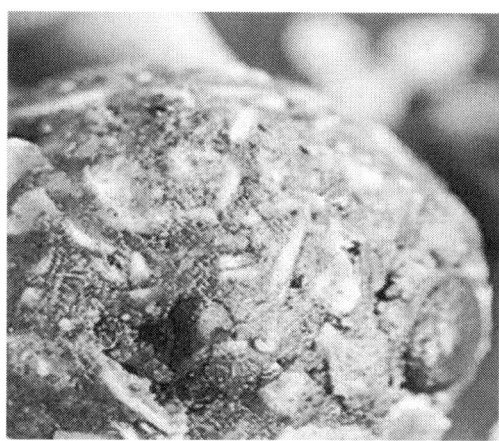

Directions

1. Mix up together the whisked egg, almond milk, apple cider vinegar, baking powder, vanilla extract, and butter.
2. Stir the mixture and add almond flour and coconut flakes. Knead the dough.
3. If the dough is sticky – add more almond flour.
4. Make the medium balls from the dough and place them on the rack of Ninja Foodi.
5. Press them gently with the hand palm.
6. Lower the air fryer lid and cook the dessert for 12 minutes at 360 F.
7. Check if the dessert is cooked – and cook for 2 minutes more for a crunchy crust.
8. Enjoy!

Nutritional Information: Calories: 118, Fat: 11.5g, Carbohydrates: 2.4g, Protein: 2.7g

Ginger Cookies

Servings: 7

Preparation Time: 25 minutes

Ingredients

- 1 cup almond flour
- 3 tablespoons butter
- 1 egg
- ½ teaspoon baking powder
- 3 tablespoon Erythritol
- 1 teaspoon ground ginger
- ½ teaspoon ground cinnamon
- 3 tablespoons heavy cream

Directions

1. Beat the egg in the bowl and whisk it gently.
2. Add baking powder, Erythritol, ground ginger, ground cinnamon, heavy cream, and flour. Stir gently and add butter,
3. Knead the non-sticky dough. Roll up the dough with the help of the rolling pin and make the cookies with the help of the cutter.
4. Place the cookies in the basket in one layer and close the lid.
5. Set the Bake mode and cook the cookies for 14 minutes at 350 F.
6. When the cookies are cooked – let them chill well and serve!

Nutritional Information: Calories: 172, Fat: 15.6g, Carbohydrates: 4.1g, Protein: 4.4g

Mini Cheese Cakes

Servings: 4

Preparation Time: 35 minutes

Ingredients

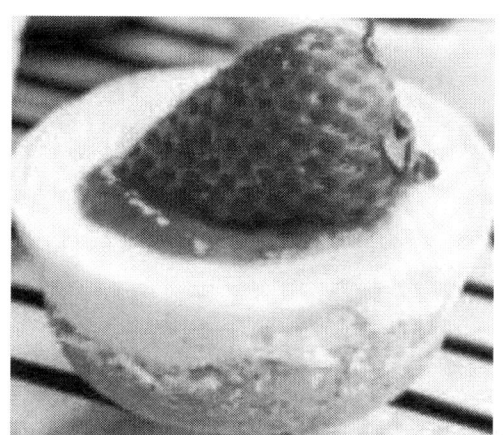

- 8 tablespoons cream cheese
- 4 tablespoon Erythritol
- 2 tablespoons heavy cream
- ½ teaspoon vanilla extract
- 4 tablespoons almond flour

Directions

1. Whisk together the cream cheese and heavy cream.
2. When the mixture is smooth – add 1 tablespoon of Erythritol and stir until homogenous.
3. After this, add vanilla extract and stir again.
4. Scoop the medium balls from the cream cheese mixture.
5. Mix up together the almond flour and all the remaining Erythritol.
6. Then coat every cheesecake ball into the almond flour mixture.
7. Freeze the balls for 20 minutes or until they are solid.
8. Place the cheesecake balls in the Ninja Foodi basket and lower the air fryer lid. Cook the dessert at 400 F for 4 minutes.
9. When the time is over – serve the dessert immediately.

Nutritional Information: Calories: 139, Fat: 13.1g, Carbohydrates: 2.3g, Protein: 3.2g

Vanilla Crème Brulee

Servings: 3

Preparation Time: 30 minutes

Ingredients

- 1 cup heavy cream
- 4 egg yolks
- 3 tablespoons Truvia
- ½ teaspoon vanilla extract

Directions

1. Whisk together the egg yolks and 2 tablespoons of Truvia.
2. Add heavy cream and stir until homogenous.
3. Place the mixture into the ramekins and cover them with the foil
4. Make the small holes on the top of the foil with the help of the toothpick.
5. Pour ½ cup of water in Ninja foodi basket and insert trivet
6. Place the ramekins on the trivet and close the pressure cooker lid
7. Cook the dessert on Pressure mode (High Pressure) for 10 minutes. Then make quick pressure release for 5 minutes.
8. Let the dessert chill for 10 minutes.
9. Remove the foil from the ramekins and sprinkle the surface of crème brulee with Truvia
10. Use the hand torch to caramelize the surface.
11. Serve!

Nutritional Information: Calories: 139, Fat: 13.1g, Carbohydrates: 2.3g, Protein: 3.2g

Delicious Lemon Mousse

Servings: 2

Preparation Time: 25 minutes

Ingredients

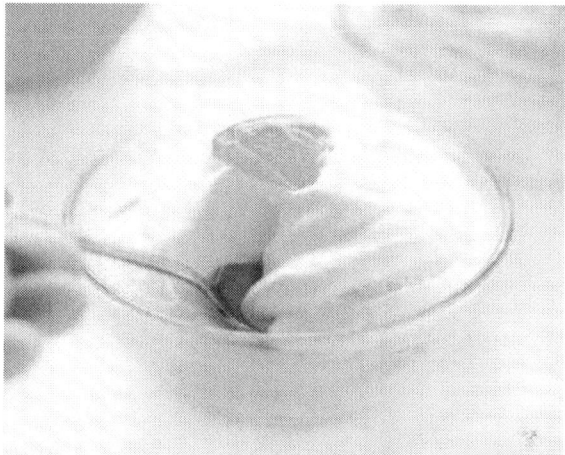

- 1-2 ounces cream cheese, soft
- ½ cup heavy cream
- 1/8 cup fresh lemon juice
- ½ teaspoon lemon liquid stevia
- 2 pinch salt

Directions

1. Take a bowl and mix in cream cheese, heavy cream, lemon juice, salt and stevia
2. Pour the mixture into ramekins and transfer the ramekins to your Ninja Foodi pot
3. Lock lid and select "Bake/Roast" mode and bake for 12 minutes at 350 degrees F
4. Pour the mixture into

Nutritional Information (per serving): Calories: 292, Fat: 26g, Carbohydrates: 8g, Protein: 5g

Cinnamon Bun

Servings: 8

Preparation Time: 25 minutes

Ingredients

- 1 cup almond flour
- ½ teaspoon baking powder
- 3 tablespoon Erythritol
- 2 tablespoon ground cinnamon
- ½ teaspoon vanilla extract
- 1 tablespoon butter
- 1 egg, whisked
- ¾ teaspoon salt
- ¼ cup almond milk

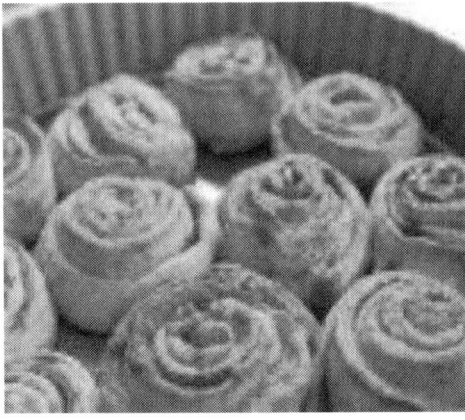

Directions

1. Mix up together the almond flour, baking powder, vanilla extract, egg, salt, and almond milk.
2. Knead the soft and non-sticky dough.
3. Roll up the dough with the help of the rolling pin
4. Sprinkle dough with the butter, cinnamon, and Erythritol.
5. Roll the dough into the log.
6. Cut the roll into 7 pieces.
7. Spray Ninja foodi basket with the cooking spray.
8. Place the cinnamon buns in the basket and close the lid.
9. Set the Bake mode and cook the buns for 15 minutes at 355F
10. Check if the buns are cooked with the help of the toothpick.
11. Chill the buns well and serve!

Nutritional Information: Calories: 292, Fat: 26g, Carbohydrates: 8g, Protein: 5g

Pumpkin Muffins

Servings: 5

Preparation Time: 27 minutes

Ingredients

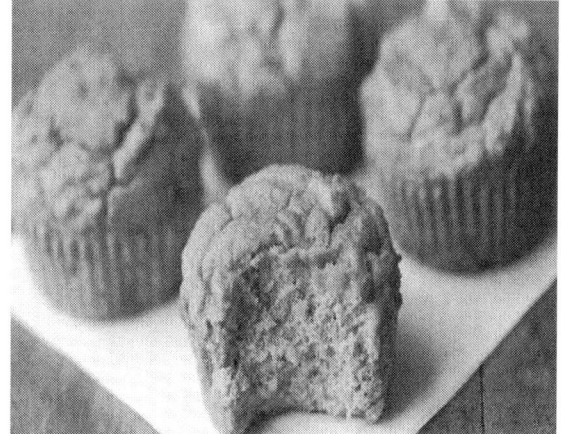

- 1 tablespoon butter, melted
- 1 tablespoon pumpkin puree
- 1 teaspoon ground cinnamon
- ¼ teaspoon ground ginger
- 1 egg, beaten
- 3 tablespoon Erythritol
- ½ cup almond flour
- ½ teaspoon baking powder

Directions

1. Mix up together all the ingredients in the mixing bowl.
2. Stir the mixture well until smooth. Transfer the mixture into the silicon muffin molds and place on the track in Ninja foodi.
3. Lower the air fryer lid and set on Bake mode
4. Cook the muffins for 20 minutes at 330 F
5. When the time is over, let the muffins rest a little and serve!

Nutritional Information: Calories: 52, Fat: 4.6g, Carbohydrates: 8.7g, Protein: 1.8g

Chocolate Cakes

Servings: 2

Preparation Time: 35 minutes

Ingredients

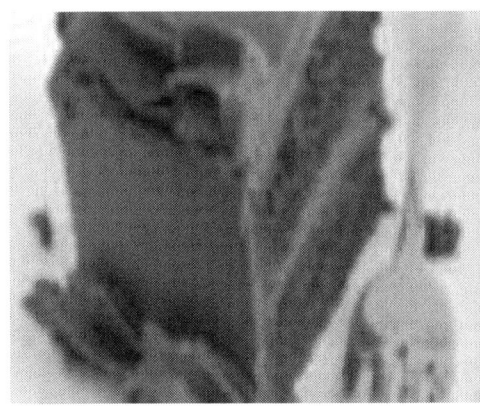

- 1 tablespoon cocoa powder
- 4 tablespoons almond flour
- ½ teaspoon vanilla extract
- 1 tablespoon Truvia
- 1/3 cup heavy cream
- ¼ teaspoon baking powder
- Cooking spray

Directions

1. Mix up together the cocoa powder, almond flour, vanilla extract, Truvia, heavy cream, and baking powder.
2. Use the mixer to make the smooth batter.
3. Spray the silicon molds with the cooking spray inside.
4. Pour the batter into the silicon molds and transfer then in Ninja foodi basket
5. Close the air fryer lid and set Bake-Roast option
6. Cook the cakes at 255 F for 22 minutes.
7. Serve the dessert chilled!

Nutritional Information: Calories: 108, Fat: 9.6g, Carbohydrates: 5.2g, Protein: 2.6g

Keto Donuts

Servings: 5

Preparation Time: 20 minutes

Ingredients

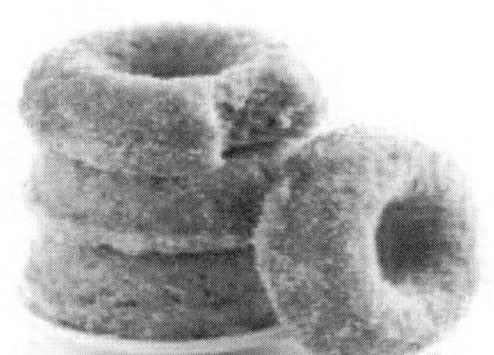

- 1 ½ cup almond flour
- ½ teaspoon baking soda
- 1 teaspoon vanilla extract
- 1 egg, whisked
- 2 tablespoons Erythritol
- ½ cup heavy cream

Directions

1. Mix up together the whisked egg, heavy cream, Erythritol, vanilla extract, and baking soda.
2. When the mixture is homogenous – add almond flour. Stir well and knead the non-sticky dough.
3. Let the dough rest for 10 minutes. After this, roll up the dough with the help of the rolling pin into 1 inch thick.
4. Then make the donuts with the help of the cutter.
5. Set the Ninja Foodi Bake mode + Roast option and set 360 F.
6. When the appliance is preheated – place the donuts in the basket and lower the air fryer lid.
7. Cook the donuts for 5 minutes.
8. Chill the donuts well and serve!

Nutritional Information: Calories: 118, Fat: 11.5g, Carbohydrates: 2.4g, Protein: 2.7g

Keto Brownie

Servings: 6

Preparation Time: 40 minutes

Ingredients

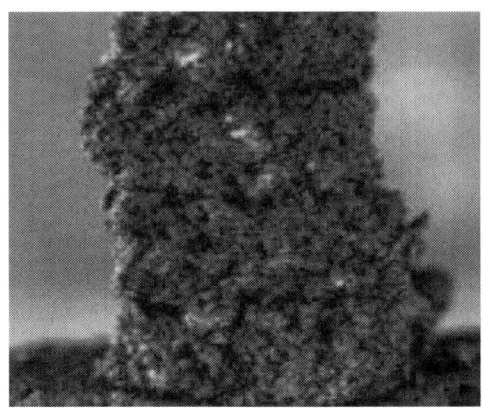

- 3 tablespoons Truvia
- 1 oz sugar-free chocolate chips
- 2 eggs, whisked
- ½ teaspoon vanilla extract
- 3 tablespoon butter, melted
- 1 tablespoon almond flour

Directions

1. Whisk together the melted butter, almond flour, vanilla extract, and Truvia.
2. Melt the chocolate chips and add them in the butter mixture.
3. Add eggs and stir until smooth.
4. Pour the batter into Ninja Foodi basket (Bake mode) and cook at 360 F for 32 minutes.
5. Then check if the brownie cooked and chill well. Cut it into the servings and serve!

Nutritional Information: Calories: 99, Fat: 8.8g, Carbohydrates: 5.9g, Protein: 2.4g

Pumpkin Pie

Servings: 4

Preparation Time: 35 minutes

Ingredients

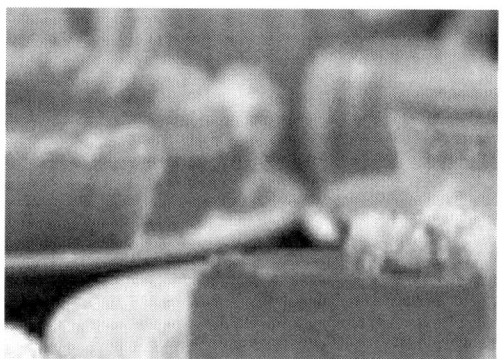

- 1 tablespoon pumpkin puree
- 1 cup coconut flour
- ½ teaspoon baking powder
- 1 teaspoon apple cider vinegar
- 1 teaspoon Pumpkin spices
- 1 tablespoon butter
- ¼ cup heavy cream
- 2 tablespoon liquid stevia
- 1 egg, whisked

Directions

1. Melt the butter and combine it together with the heavy cream, apple cider vinegar, liquid stevia, egg, and baking powder.
2. Add pumpkin puree and coconut flour.
3. After this, add pumpkin spices and stir the batter until smooth.
4. Pour the batter in Ninja Foodi basket and lower the air fryer lid.
5. Set the "Bake" mode 360 F.
6. Cook the pie for 25 minutes.
7. When the time is over – let the pie chill till the room temperature. Serve it!

Nutritional Information: Calories: 127, Fat: 6.6g, Carbohydrates: 14.2g, Protein: 3.8g

Hearty Carrot Pumpkin Pudding

Servings: 4

Preparation Time: 25 minutes

Ingredients

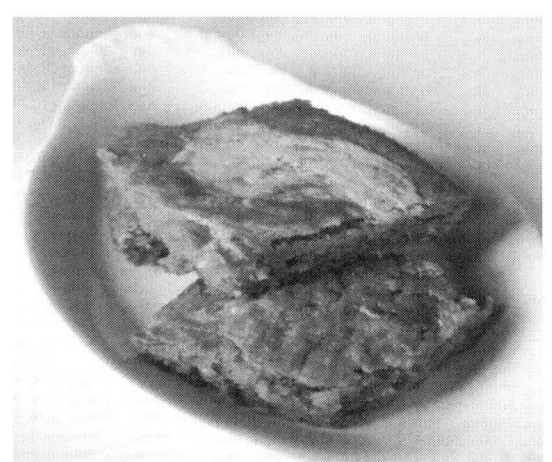

- 1 tablespoon extra-virgin olive oil
- 2 cups carrots, shredded
- 2 cups pureed pumpkin
- ½ sweet onion, finely chopped
- 1 cup heavy whip cream
- ½ cup cream cheese, soft
- 2 whole eggs
- 1 tablespoon granulated Erythritol
- 1 teaspoon ground nutmeg
- ½ teaspoon salt
- ¼ cup pumpkin seeds, garnish
- ¼ cup water

Directions

1. Add oil to your Ninja Foodi pot and whisk in carrots, pumpkin, onion, heavy cream, cream cheese, eggs, Erythritol, nutmeg, salt and water
2. Stir and lock lid
3. Cook on HIGH pressure for 10 minutes
4. Release pressure naturally over 10 minutes
5. Serve with a topping of pumpkin seeds
6. Enjoy!

Nutritional Information: Calories: 239, Fat: 19g, Carbohydrates: 7g, Protein: 6g

Mariana Cleff

Artichoke Dip

Servings: 6

Preparation Time: 8 minutes

Ingredients

- ¼ cup chicken broth
- 4 oz cream cheese
- 5 ounces chopped spinach
- 1 cup canned artichoke hearts
- ½ cup sour cream
- 1 clove garlic
- ½ tsp onion powder
- 6 ounces parmesan cheese, grated
- 6 ounces Swiss cheese

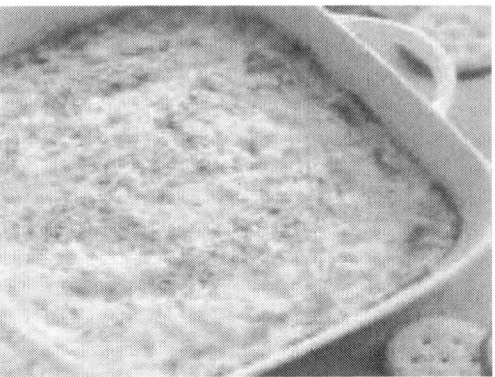

Directions:

1. Add all the ingredients to the Ninja Foodi Pot except the parmesan cheese and Swiss cheese.
2. Close the lid and set the steamer valve to seal. Use the pressure cooker function and cook the dip on high pressure for 4 minutes. Do a quick pressure release and open the pot.
3. Add the cheeses, reserving a small amount of each, and mix. Sprinkle the final cheese over the top of the dip and lower the crisper plate over the dip. Use the broil function for 2 minutes to brown the cheese.
4. Serve hot!

Nutritional Information: Calories: 72, Fat: 6g, Carbohydrates: 5g, Protein: 5g

Loaded Nachos

Servings: 4

Preparation Time: minutes

Ingredients

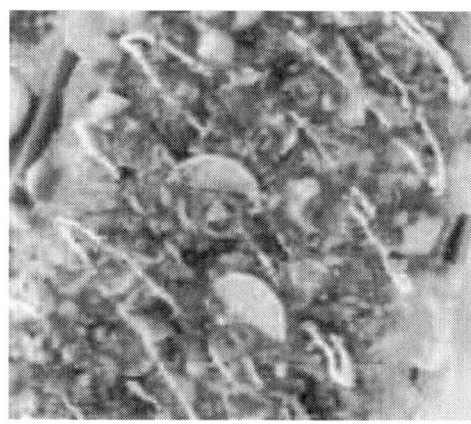

- 2 chicken breasts, boneless and skinless
- 1 cup keto salsa
- 1 tsp salt
- 1 Tbsp taco seasoning
- 4 cups grain free tortilla chips
- 1 cup shredded Mexican cheese blend
- 1 jalapeno, sliced

Directions:

1. Place the chicken and salsa in the Ninja Foodi and place the lid on as well.
2. Set the pressure cooker steam valve to seal and cook on high pressure for 15 minutes. Do a quick pressure release and remove the lid. Use two forks to shred the chicken, mixing it into the sauce.
3. Add the taco seasoning and salt to the mix and stir to combine.
4. Place the tortilla chips on top of the chicken mix inside the pot.
5. Sprinkle the shredded cheese and jalapenos over the top of the chips then close the crisper lid and set the temperature for 360 degrees for 5 minutes.
6. Remove the perfectly browned nachos and serve while warm!

Nutritional Information: Calories: 198, Fat: 10g, Carbohydrates: 3g, Protein: 5g

Buffalo Cauliflower Bites

Servings: 4

Preparation Time: 50 minutes

Ingredients

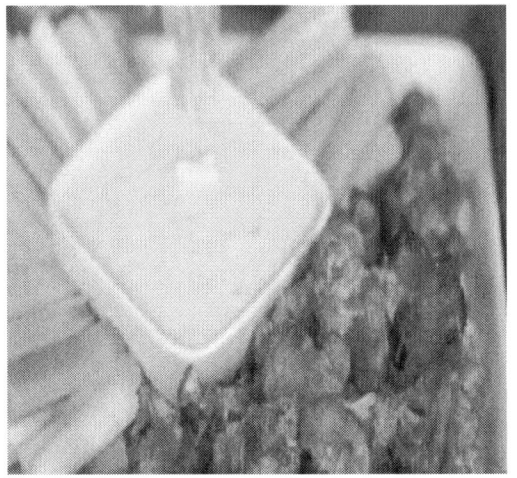

- 6 cups Cauliflower florets
- 1 ½ cups water
- 1/3 cup hot sauce
- 1 ½ cups cornstarch
- ½ cup almond flour
- 2 tsp baking powder
- 1 tsp garlic powder
- 1 tsp salt
- ½ tsp black pepper
- 2 eggs

Directions:

1. Add the cauliflower and ½ cup of the water to the bowl of the Ninja Foodi.
2. Place the lid on the machine and use the pressure cooker on low pressure to cook the cauliflower for 2 minutes. Once the cooking is complete, do a quick pressure release, and remove the lid. Cool the cauliflower in the fridge.
3. In a small bowl, mix together the corn starch, almond flour, baking powder, garlic powder, salt, eggs and pepper.
4. Add the remaining cup of water and mix until smooth. Toss the chilled cauliflower in the batter then place the coated cauliflower on a separate tray and cool in the freezer for about 30 minutes.
5. Place the chilled cauliflower in the cook and crisp basket in one layer, try not to overlap. Preheat the Ninja Foodi using the air crisp setting to 350 degrees.

6. Place the cauliflower basket into the Ninja Foodi and close the crisper lid. Set the timer to twenty minutes. Remove the cauliflower once cooked and toss with the hot sauce.
7. Serve immediately.

Nutritional Information: Calories: 72, Fat: 6g, Carbohydrates: 5g, Protein: 5g

Jicama Fries

Servings: 4

Preparation Time: 15 minutes

Ingredients

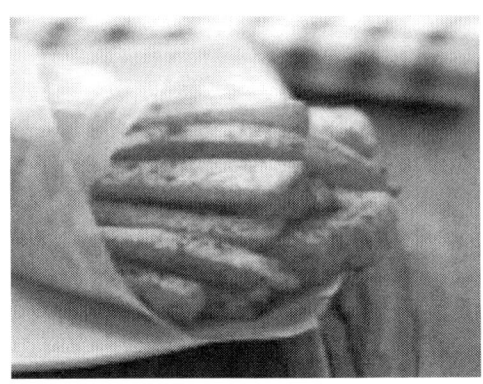

- 1 medium jicama
- 3 Tbsp olive oil
- ½ tsp salt
- ¼ tsp ground black pepper

Directions:

1. Peel the jicama and cup it into ¼ inch strips. Toss the slices with the oil, salt and pepper.
2. Place the strips in the air crisp basket, put the basket into the Ninja Foodie and put the air crisp lid on the machine.
3. Set the temperature to 390 degrees F and the timer for 20 minutes. Toss the fries occasionally to brown evenly.
4. Serve hot

Nutritional Information: Calories: 101, Fat: 10g, Carbohydrates: 3g, Protein: 0g

The Original Pot-De-Crème

Servings: 4

Preparation Time: 30 minutes

Ingredients

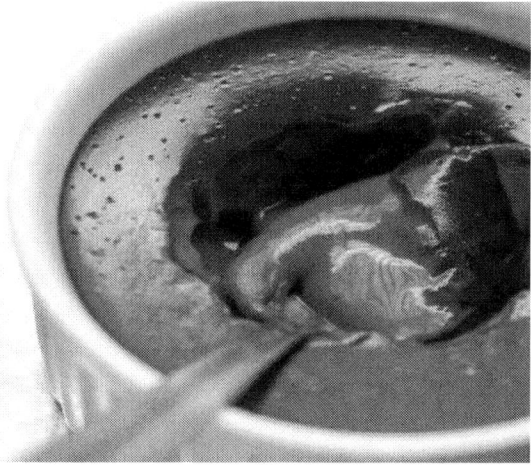

- 6 egg yolks
- 2 cups heavy whip cream
- 1/3 cup cocoa powder
- 1 tablespoon pure vanilla extract
- ½ teaspoon liquid stevia
- Whipped coconut cream as needed for garnish
- Shaved dark chocolate, for garnish

Directions

1. Take a medium bowl and whisk in yolks, heavy cream, cocoa powder, vanilla and stevia
2. Pour the mixture into 1 and ½ quart baking dish and place the dish in your Ninja Foodi insert
3. Add enough water to reach about halfway up the sides of baking dish
4. Lock lid and cook on HIGH pressure for 12 minutes
5. Quick release pressure once the cycle is complete
6. Remove baking dish from insert and let it cool
7. Chill the dessert in refrigerator and serve with garnish of whipped coconut cream and shaved dark chocolate
8. Enjoy!

Nutritional Information: Calories: 275, Fat: 18g, Carbohydrates: 3g, Protein: 5g

Chapter Seven: Keto Ninja Foodi Vegan and Vegetarian

Cauliflower Puree with Scallions

Serves: 6

Preparation time: 20 minutes

Ingredients

- 1 head cauliflower
- 4 cups of water
- 1 tablespoon salt
- 4 tablespoons butter
- 3 ounces scallions
- 1 teaspoon chicken stock
- ¼ teaspoon sesame seeds
- 1 egg yolk

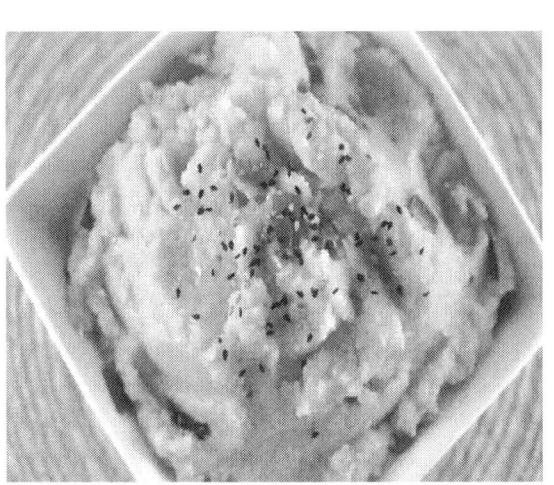

Directions:

1. Wash the cauliflower and chop it roughly. Place the cauliflower in the pressure cooker. Add the water and salt.
2. Close the pressure cooker lid and cook the vegetables on "Pressure" mode for 5 minutes. Release the pressure and open the pressure cooker lid. Remove the cauliflower from the pressure cooker and let it rest briefly.
3. Place the cauliflower in a blender. Add the butter, chicken stock, and sesame seeds. Blend the mixture well.
4. Chop the scallions. Add the egg yolk to the blender and blend the mixture for 30 seconds.
5. Remove the cauliflower puree from the blender and combine it with the scallions. Mix well and serve.

Nutritional Information: calories 94, fat 8.7g, carbs 3.39g, protein 2g

Garlic and Dill Carrot Fiesta

Servings: 4

Preparation Time: 12 minutes

Ingredients

- 3 cups carrots, chopped
- 1 tablespoon melted butter
- ½ teaspoon garlic sea salt
- 1 tablespoon fresh dill, minced
- 1 cup water

Directions

1. Add listed ingredients to Ninja Foodi
2. Stir and lock lid, cook on HIGH pressure for 10 minutes
3. Release pressure naturally over 10 minutes
4. Quick release pressure and remove lid
5. Serve with a topping of dill, enjoy!

Nutritional Information: Calories: 207, Fat: 16g, Carbohydrates: 5g, Protein: 8g

Zucchini Gratin

Servings: 6

Preparation Time: 13 minutes

Ingredients

- 2 zucchini, sliced
- 1 cup cream cheese
- 4 oz Cheddar cheese, shredded
- 1 teaspoon ground black pepper
- 1 teaspoon salt
- ¼ cup fresh dill chopped
- ¾ cup walnuts, chopped
- 1 teaspoon olive oil

Directions:

1. Brush the cooker basket with olive oil from inside. Make the layer of the sliced zucchini in it. Then spread it with the cream cheese and walnuts.
2. After this, add shredded cheese, salt, and dill. Then repeat the same steps until you use all the ingredients. Close the lid and cook the gratin on low-pressure mode for 3 hours.
3. Then chill the gratin till the room temperature and transfer onto the serving plates

Nutritional Information: calories 331, fat 30g, carbs 6.4g, protein 12.6g

Asian-Style Asparagus and Tofu Scramble

Serves: 2

Preparation Time: 15 minutes

Ingredients

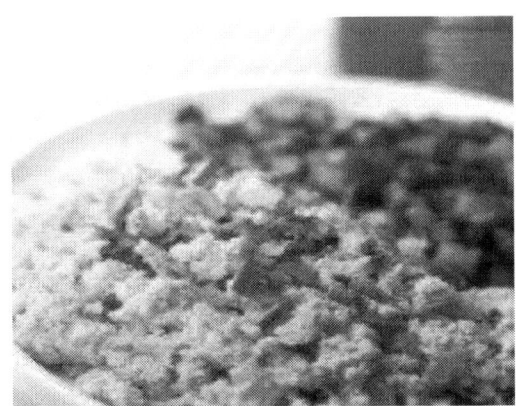

- 1 tablespoon sesame oil
- 10 ounces soft silken tofu, drained and chopped
- 6 ounces asparagus
- 2 garlic cloves, finely minced
- 1 teaspoon fresh lemon juice
- 1 tablespoon soy sauce
- 1/2 teaspoon paprika
- 1/2 teaspoon coarse salt
- Freshly cracked mixed peppercorns, to taste
- 1/2 cup fresh basil, roughly chopped

Directions

1. Add 1 cup of water and a rack to the cooking pot. Place the asparagus on the rack.
2. Secure the pressure lid; press the STEAM button and cook for 2 minutes at High Pressure.
3. Once cooking is complete, use a quick release; remove the lid carefully.
4. Cut the cooked asparagus into pieces.
5. Stir in the other ingredients, except the basil leaves. Secure the crisping lid and choose the AIR CRISP function.
6. Set the temperature to 380 degrees F and set the time to 10 minutes; press the START/STOP button.
7. Serve warm garnished with fresh basil leaves. Bon appétit!

Nutritional Information: Calories 160, Carbs 8.5g, Fats 10.8g, Protein 8.9g

Zucchini Pizza

Preparation time: 18 minutes

Servings: 2

Ingredients

- 1 zucchini
- ½ teaspoon tomato paste
- 5 oz Parmesan, shredded
- ½ teaspoon chili flakes
- ¼ teaspoon dried basil
- 1 teaspoon olive oil

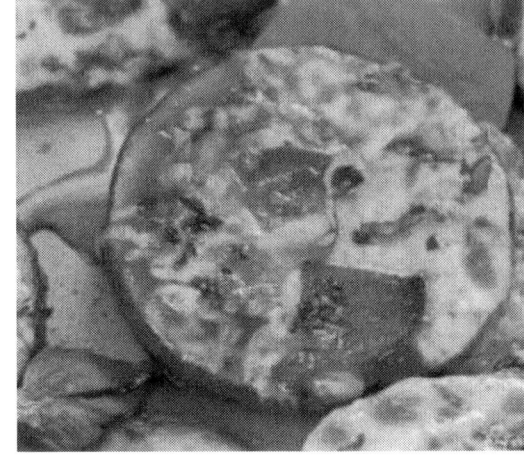

Directions:

1. Cut the zucchini into halves to get boards. Then scoop the flesh from them and spread with the tomato paste from inside.
2. After this, fill zucchini with the shredded cheese. Sprinkle them with chili flakes, dried basil, and olive oil.
3. Put the zucchini pizzas in the cooker and close the lid. Cook the pizzas on air crisp mode at 375F for 8 minutes.

Nutritional Information: calories 331, fat 21.9g, carbs 6g, protein 28.1g

Steamed Kale

Serves: 6

Preparation time: 16 minutes

Ingredients

- 1-pound kale
- 1 teaspoon garlic powder
- 1 teaspoon olive oil
- ¾ cup heavy cream
- 1 tablespoon almonds, chopped
- 1 teaspoon salt
- 1 cup water, for cooking

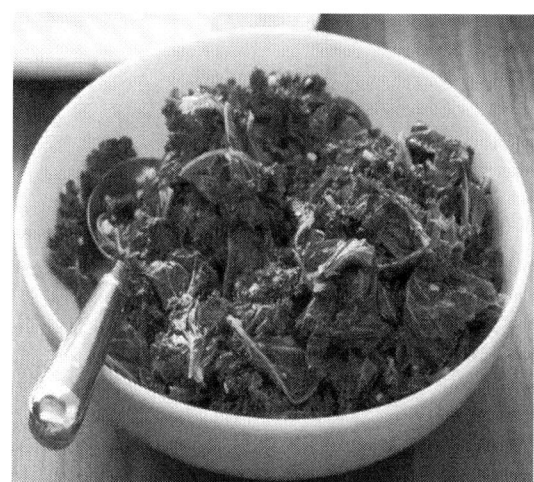

Directions:

1. Chop the kale roughly. Pour water in the cooker and insert trivet.
2. Place the chopped kale on the trivet. Close the lid and steam the greens for 6 minutes.
3. Meanwhile, mix up together olive oil, cream almonds, and salt. When the kale is cooked, transfer it into the serving bowls and sprinkle with the heavy cream mixture.

Nutritional Information: calories 103, fat 6.8g, carbs 8.9g, protein 2.9g

Quinoa with Veggies

Serves: 6

Preparation Time: 20 minutes

Ingredients

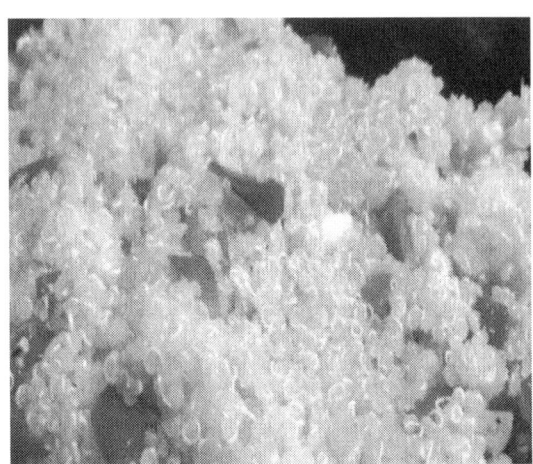

- 2 cups quinoa
- 4 cups vegetable stock
- 2 onions, chopped
- 1 head broccoli, chopped into small-sized florets
- 2 ripe tomatoes, chopped
- 3 cloves garlic, finely minced
- 3 teaspoons canola oil
- 1/2 teaspoon ground black pepper
- 1 teaspoon dried basil
- 1 teaspoon kosher salt
- 1/4 cup chopped fresh chives, for garnish

Directions

1. Add the quinoa and vegetable stock to the Ninja Foodi.
2. Secure the pressure lid; press the PRESSURE button and cook for 1 minute at High Pressure. Once cooking is complete, use a natural release; remove the lid carefully. Place the rack over the quinoa.
3. Place the rest of the above ingredients on the rack, except for the chives.
4. Secure the crisping lid and choose the BAKE/ROAST function.
5. Set the temperature to 390 degrees F and set the time to 10 minutes; press the START/STOP button. Taste and adjust the seasonings.
6. Sprinkle with fresh chives and serve.

Nutritional Information: Calories 160, Carbs 8.5g, Fats 10.8g, Protein 8.9g

Roasted Green Beans with Lime Juice

Serves: 4

Preparation Time: 25 mins

Ingredients

- 1 ½ tablespoons dark sesame oil
- 1/2 teaspoon cayenne pepper
- 10 ounces green beans, canned and drained
- 1 teaspoon ground cumin
- 1 teaspoon chili powder
- Salt and ground black pepper, to taste
- 1 ½ tablespoons lime juice

Directions

1. Add 1 ½ cups of a lightly salted water and green beans to the inner cooking pot.
2. Secure the pressure lid; press the PRESSURE button and cook for 1 minute at Low Pressure.
3. Once cooking is complete, use a quick release; remove the lid carefully.
4. Now, drain the green beans and dry them on a kitchen towel.
5. Toss the green beans with the remaining ingredients until evenly coated.
6. Add the green beans to the cooking basket; place the cooking basket in your Ninja Foodi.
7. Secure the crisping lid and choose the AIR CRISP function.
8. Set the temperature to 380F and set the time to 5 minutes; press the START/STOP button. Enjoy!

Nutritional Information: Calories 68, Carbs 4.5g, Fats 5.4g, Protein 0.7g

Hot and Spicy Black Beans

Serves: 5

Preparation Time: 40 mins

Ingredients

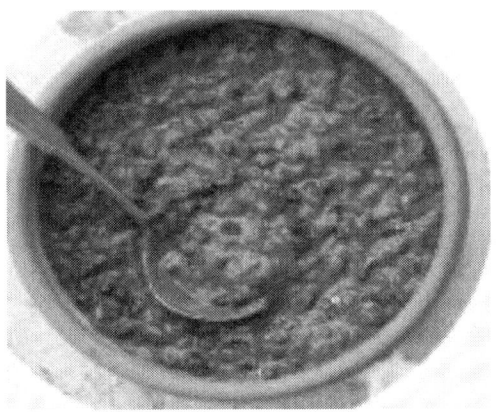

- 2 tablespoons olive oil
- 2 red onions, diced
- 3 cloves garlic, smashed
- 1 bell pepper, chopped
- 1/2 teaspoon ancho chili pepper, minced
- 2 cups tomatoes, puréed
- 1 ¼ pounds dry black beans, rinsed and drained
- 2 cups vegetable broth
- Morton kosher salt and ground black pepper, to taste
- 1 teaspoon cayenne pepper
- 2 bay leaves
- 2 tablespoons fresh cilantro leaves, roughly chopped

Directions

1. Press the SEAR/SAUTÉ button and set to Medium-High.
2. Once hot, heat the oil and sauté the onions until tender and aromatic.
3. Then, add the garlic and peppers; cook an additional 1 minute 30 seconds or until fragrant.
4. After that, stir the puréed tomatoes, black beans, broth, salt, black pepper, cayenne pepper, and bay leaves into the cooking pot.
5. Secure the pressure lid; press the PRESSURE button and cook for 12 minutes at High Pressure.
6. Once cooking is complete, use a natural release; remove the lid carefully.

7. Secure the crisping lid and choose the BAKE/ROAST function. Set the temperature to 370F and set the time to 12 minutes; press the START/STOP button.
8. Garnish with fresh cilantro leaves and serve.

Nutritional Information: Calories 276, Carbs 4.5g, Fats 5.4g, Protein 0.7g

Astounding Caramelized Onions

Servings: 4

Preparation Time: 55 minutes

Ingredients

- 2 tablespoons unsalted butter
- 3 large onions, sliced
- 2 tablespoons water
- 1 teaspoon salt

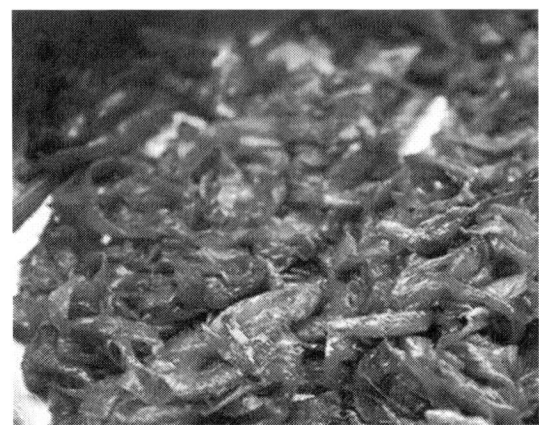

Directions

1. Set your pot to Sauté mode and adjust the heat to Medium, pre-heat the inner pot for 5 minutes
2. Add butter and let it melt, add onions, water, salt, and stir well
3. Lock pressure lid into place, making sure that the pressure valve is locked
4. Cook on HIGH pressure for 30 minutes
5. Quick release the pressure once done
6. Remove the lid and set the pot to Sauté mode, let it sear in the Medium-HIGH mode for about 15 minutes until the liquid is almost gone
7. Enjoy!

Nutritional Information: Calories: 110, Fat: 6g, Carbohydrates: 10g, Protein: 2g

Herb Carrots

Servings: 5

Preparation Time: 30 minutes

Ingredients

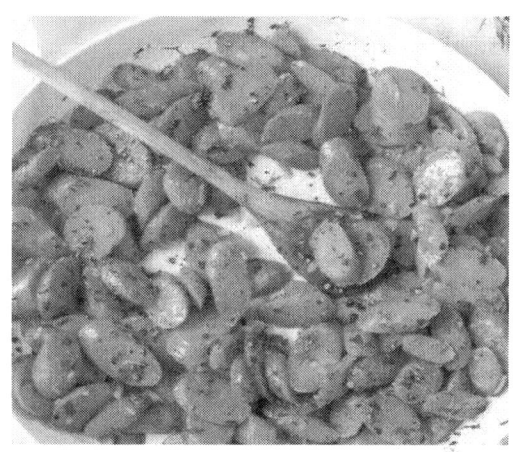

- 1-pound carrots
- 1 teaspoon salt
- 1 teaspoon cilantro
- ½ teaspoon ground ginger
- 1 teaspoon paprika
- 1 tablespoon basil
- ¼ teaspoon rosemary
- ⅓ cup half and half
- 1 teaspoon minced garlic
- 1 teaspoon white pepper

Directions

1. Peel the carrots and cut them into bite-sized pieces.
2. Combine the salt, cilantro, ground ginger, paprika, basil, white pepper, and rosemary together in a mixing bowl. Stir the spice mixture carefully and add the carrots.
3. Set the pressure cooker to" Steam" mode.
4. Place the carrots in the trivet and place it into the pressure cooker. Cook for 20 minutes.
5. When the cooking time ends, remove the dish from the pressure cooker and transfer the carrots to a serving plate.
6. Combine the half and half with the minced garlic and mix well.
7. Pour the cream onto the carrots and serve.

Summertime Veggie Soup

Servings: 6

Preparation Time: 23 minutes

Ingredients

- 3 cups leeks, sliced
- 6 cups rainbow chard, stems and leaves, chopped
- 1 cup celery, chopped
- 2 tablespoons garlic, minced
- 1 teaspoon dried oregano
- 1 teaspoon salt
- 2 teaspoons fresh ground black pepper
- 3 cups chicken broth
- 2 cups yellow summer squash, sliced into 1/ inch slices
- ¼ cup fresh parsley, chopped
- ¾ cup heavy whip cream
- 4-6 tablespoons parmesan cheese, grated

Directions

1. Add leeks, chard, celery, 1 tablespoon garlic, oregano, salt, pepper and broth to your Ninja Foodi
2. Lock lid and cook on HIGH pressure for 3 minutes
3. Quick release pressure
4. Open lid and add more broth, set your pot to Sauté mode and adjust heat to HIGH
5. Add yellow squash, parsley and remaining 1 tablespoon garlic
6. Let it cook for 2-3 minutes until the squash is soft
7. Stir in cream and sprinkle parmesan
8. Serve

Nutritional Information: Calories: 210, Fat: 14g, Carbohydrates: 10g, Protein: 10g

Delicious Mushroom Stroganoff

Servings: 6

Preparation Time: 15 minutes

Ingredients

- ¼ cup unsalted butter, cubed
- 1-pound cremini mushrooms, halved
- 1 large onion, halved
- 4 garlic cloves, minced
- 2 cups vegetable broth
- ½ teaspoon salt
- ¼ teaspoon fresh black pepper
- 1 and ½ cups sour cream
- ¼ cup fresh flat-leaf parsley, chopped
- 1 cup grated parmesan cheese

Directions

1. Add butter, mushrooms, onion, garlic, vegetable broth, salt, pepper and paprika
2. Gently stir and lock lid
3. Cook on HIGH pressure for 5 minutes
4. Release pressure naturally over 10 minutes
5. Serve by stirring in sour cream and with a garnish of parsley and parmesan cheese

Nutritional Information: Calories: 453, Fat: 37g, Carbohydrates: 11g, Protein: 19g

Offbeat Cauliflower and Cheddar Soup

Servings: 4

Preparation Time: 16 minutes

Ingredients

- ¼ cup butter
- ½ sweet onion, chopped
- 1 head cauliflower, chopped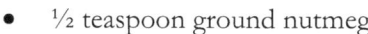
- 4 cups herbed vegetable stock
- ½ teaspoon ground nutmeg
- 1 cup heavy whip cream
- Salt and pepper as needed
- 1 cup cheddar cheese, shredded

Directions

1. Set your Ninja Foodi to sauté mode and add butter, let it heat up and melt
2. Add onion and Cauliflower, Sauté for 10 minutes until tender and lightly browned
3. Add vegetable stock and nutmeg, bring to a boil
4. Lock lid and cook on HIGH pressure for 5 minutes, quick release pressure once done
5. Remove pot and from Foodi and stir in heavy cream, puree using immersion blender
6. Season with more salt and pepper and serve with a topping of cheddar
7. Enjoy!

Nutritional Information: Calories: 227, Fat: 21g, Carbohydrates: 4g, Protein: 8g

Medi-Cheese Spinach

Servings: 4

Preparation Time: 20 minutes

Ingredients

- 4 tablespoons butter
- 2 pounds spinach, chopped and boiled
- Salt and pepper to taste
- 2/3 cup Kalamata olives, halved and pitted
- 1 and ½ cups feta cheese, grated
- 4 teaspoons fresh lemon zest, grated

Directions

1. Take a bowl and mix spinach, butter, salt, pepper and transfer the mixture to your Crisping Basket of the Ninja Foodi
2. Transfer basket to your Foodi and lock Crisping lid
3. Cook for 15 minutes on Air Crisp mode on 340 degrees F
4. Serve by stirring in olives, lemon zest and feta

Nutritional Information: Calories: 274, Fat: 18g, Carbohydrates: 6g, Protein: 10g

Butternut Squash Soup

Servings: 4

Preparation Time: 26 minutes

Ingredients

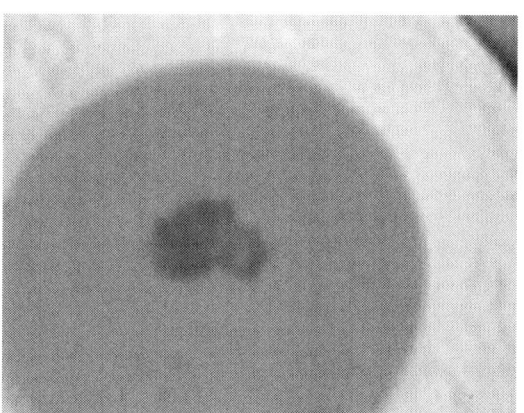

- 1 ½ pounds butternut squash, baked, peeled and cubed
- ½ cup green onions, chopped
- 3 tablespoons butter
- ½ cup carrots, peeled and chopped
- ½ cup celery, chopped
- 29 ounces vegetable stock
- 1 garlic clove, peeled and minced
- ½ teaspoon Italian seasoning
- 15 ounces canned tomatoes, diced
- Salt and pepper to taste
- 1/8 teaspoon red pepper flakes
- 1/8 teaspoon nutmeg, grated
- 1 and ½ cup half and half

Directions

1. Set your Ninja Foodi to "Sauté" mode and add butter, let it melt
2. Add celery, carrots, onion and stir cook for 3 minutes
3. Add garlic, stir cook for 1 minute
4. Add squash, tomatoes, stock, Italian seasoning, salt, pepper, pepper flakes and nutmeg, stir
5. Lock lid and cook on HIGH pressure for 10 minutes
6. Release pressure naturally over 10 minutes
7. Use an immersion blender to puree the mix

8. Set the food to Sauté mode on LOW and add half and half, stir cook for 1-2 minutes until thickened
9. Divide and serve with a sprinkle of green onions on top

Nutritional Information: Calories: 250, Fat: 22g, Carbohydrates: 8g, Protein: 3g

Zucchini Fries

Servings: 4

Preparation Time: 35 minutes

Ingredients

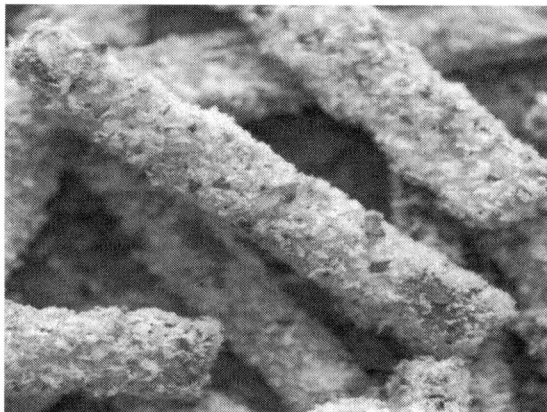

- 2 cups almond flour
- 2 Zucchinis
- 2 tsp salt
- ½ tsp ground black pepper
- 3 eggs
- 1 tbsp garlic powder
- 1 cup grated parmesan cheese
- 2 tsp onion powder

Directions

1. Cut the zucchini into strips about ¼ inch wide and 3 inches long. Sprinkle with the salt and let sit for about 20 minutes then pat dry to take any extra moisture off the fries
2. Add the almond flour and ground black pepper to a bowl and put the eggs in a separate small bowl and whisk briefly
3. In a third small bowl, mix the parmesan, garlic powder and onion powder together
4. Dip the fries one at a time in the flour then in the egg mix and finally in the cheese mix and set coated fries aside on a plate. Dip all the fries
5. Place the fries in the cook and crisp basket and then put the basket inside the pot. Lose the crisper lid and set the temperature to 375 degrees F and set the timer for 12 minutes
6. Serve fries while hot

Nutritional information: Calories: 575, Fat: 38g, Carbohydrates: 12g, Protein: 47g

Bacon and Cabbage

Servings: 4

Preparation Time: 16 minutes

Ingredients

- 3 slices bacon
- 1 head cabbage, core removed
- 4 tbsp butter
- 2 cups chicken broth
- 1 tsp salt
- ½ tsp black pepper

Directions

1. Use the sauté function to cook the bacon strips for about 8 minutes, flipping halfway through. Add the butter to the pot and stir to melt.
2. Chop the cabbage and place it into the pot with the cooked bacon
3. Add the chicken, salt and pepper to the bowl and stir to combine everything
4. Place the pressure cooker lid on the Ninja Foodie and set the steamer valve to seal. Pressure cook for three minutes on high heat then quickly release the steam by opening the steamer valve carefully.
5. Serve the bacon cabbage while hot

Nutritional Information: Calories: 236, Fat: 14g, Carbohydrates: 1g, Protein: 5g

Spicy Green Beans

Servings: 4

Preparation Time: 20 minutes

Ingredients

- 1 tbsp coconut oil
- 1-pound green beans, ends trimmed
- 1 tsp coconut aminos
- 1 tsp rice wine vinegar
- 1 garlic clove, chopped
- ¾ tsp red pepper flakes

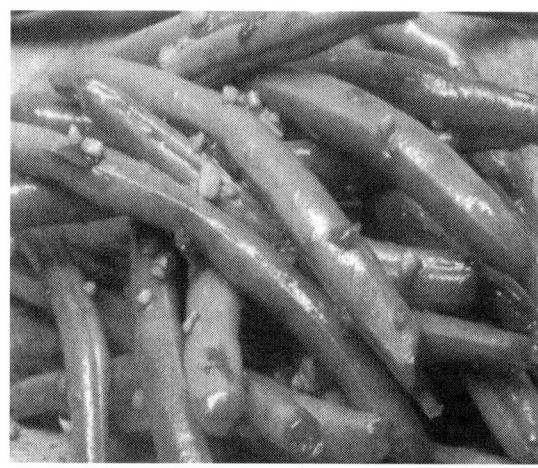

Directions

1. Toss all the ingredients together in a bowl and let sit for 10 minutes to marinate
2. Add the green beans into the crisp and cook basket and set the air crisper to 400 degrees F for 10 minutes
3. Remove the green beans and serve hot

Nutritional Information: Calories: 69, Fat: 4g, Carbohydrates: 9g, Protein: 2g

Kale Chips

Servings: 4

Preparation Time: 15minutes

Ingredients

- ¼ tsp garlic powder
- 1 bunch curly leaf kale, chopped, steams removed
- 1 bunch curly leaf kale
- ¼ tsp baking stevia
- 3 tbsp olive oil
- 1 ½ tsp salt

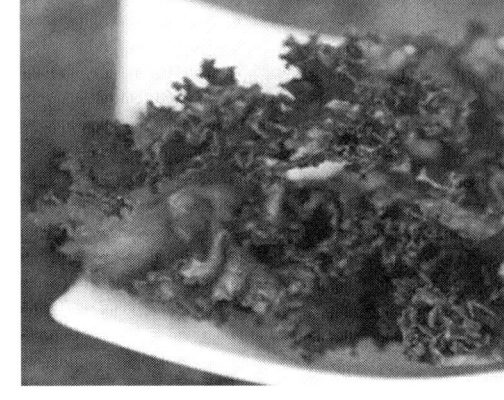

Directions

1. Toss the kale leaves in the olive oil and then add the dry seasonings and toss again
2. Place the kale on a dehydrating rack inside the Ninja Foodi, being careful not to overlap the leaves too much.
3. Place the lid on the Foodi and set the dehydrator function to 135 degrees for 7 hours
4. Remove the lid once the time has completed and allow the chips to cool. Store in an air tight container

Nutritional Information: Calories: 108, Fat: 10g, Carbohydrates: 2g, Protein: 1g

Chapter Eight: Keto Ninja Foodi Seafood Recipes

Herby Cods

Servings: 4

Preparation Time: 13 minutes

Ingredients

- 4 garlic cloves, minced
- 2 teaspoons coconut aminos
- ¼ cup butter
- 6 whole eggs
- 2 small onions, chopped
- 3 (4 ounces each) skinless cod fish fillets, cut into rectangular pieces
- 2 green chilies, chopped
- Salt and pepper to taste

Directions

1. Take a shallow dish and add all ingredients except cod, beat the mixture well
2. Dip each fillet into the mixture and keep it on the side
3. Transfer prepared fillets to your Ninja Foodi Crisping basket and transfer basket to Pot
4. Lock Crisping lid and cook on "Air Crisp" mode for 8 minutes at 330 degrees F
5. Serve!

Nutritional Information: Calories: 409, Fat: 25g, Carbohydrates: 7g, Protein: 37g

Salmon and Balsamic Shallots

Servings: 2

Preparation Time: 17 minutes

Ingredients

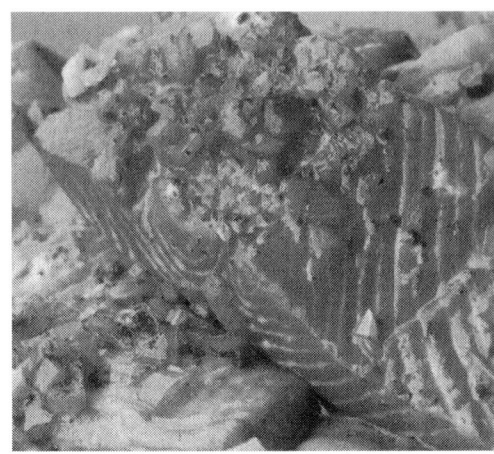

- 2 salmon fillets; boneless
- 1/3 cup balsamic vinegar
- 4 shallots; chopped.
- 2 tablespoons organic essential olive oil
- 2 tablespoon lime juice
- Salt and black pepper around the taste

Directions

1. Set the Foodi on Sauté mode, add the oil, heat it down, add the shallots and sauté them for 4 minutes.
2. Add the lime juice, vinegar, salt and pepper, toss and cook for just two minutes more.
3. Add the salmon, place pressure to succeed lid on and cook everything on High for ten mins.
4. Release pressure to ensure success fast for 5 minutes, divide between plates and serve.

Nutritional Information: Calories: 302, Fat: 12g, Carbohydrates: 7.6g, Protein: 36.6g

Marjoram Salmon

Servings: 4

Preparation Time: 13 minutes

Ingredients

- 1-pound salmon fillet
- 1 tablespoon marjoram
- ½ teaspoon rosemary
- 1 tablespoons salt
- ½ cup dill
- 1 cup of water
- 1 teaspoon cilantro
- 1 tablespoon paprika
- 1 teaspoon butter
- 1 teaspoon onion powder

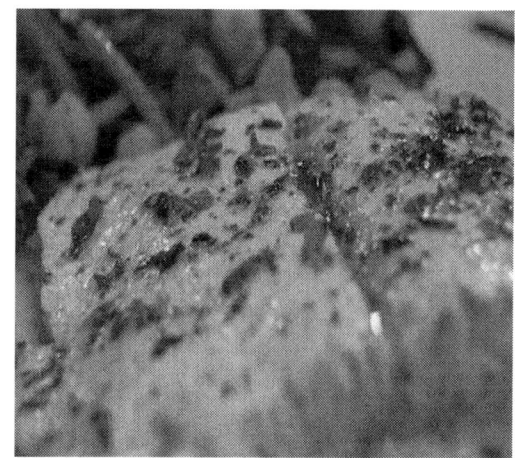

Directions

1. Combine the marjoram, rosemary, and salt in a small bowl. Rub the salmon fillet with the spice mixture.
2. Chop the dill and combine it with the onion powder and paprika in a mixing bowl. Add cilantro and stir well.
3. Place the salmon fillet on the steamer rack and transfer it to the pressure cooker. Set the pressure cooker to" Steam" mode.
4. Sprinkle the salmon with the dill mixture. Close the pressure cooker and cook the fish for 15 minutes.
5. When the cooking time ends, release the remaining pressure and let the salmon rest briefly.
6. Transfer the dish to a serving plate.

Nutritional Information: Calories: 127, Fat: 6.2g, Carbohydrates:1.17g, Protein: 16g

Tender Octopus

Servings: 6

Preparation time: 20 minutes

Ingredients:

- 1 teaspoon salt
- 10 ounces octopus
- 1 teaspoon cilantro
- 2 tablespoons olive oil
- 1 teaspoon garlic powder
- 1 teaspoon lime juice
- 1cup of water

Directions:

1. Place the octopus into the pressure cooker. Sprinkle it with the cilantro, garlic powder, and salt and mix well.
2. Add the water into the pressure cooker and close the lid. Set the pressure cooker to "Pressure" mode. Cook the dish on for 8 minutes.
3. Remove the dish from the pressure cooker and put in the tray filled with the octopus. Sprinkle the seafood with olive oil.
4. Preheat the oven to 360 F and transfer the tray to the oven. Cook the dish for 7 minutes. When the octopus is cooked, remove it from the oven and sprinkle with lemon juice. Let it rest briefly before serving.

Nutritional Information: calories 80, fat 5g, carbs 1.49g, protein 7g

Fish Curry

Servings: 5

Preparation Time: 20 minutes

Ingredients

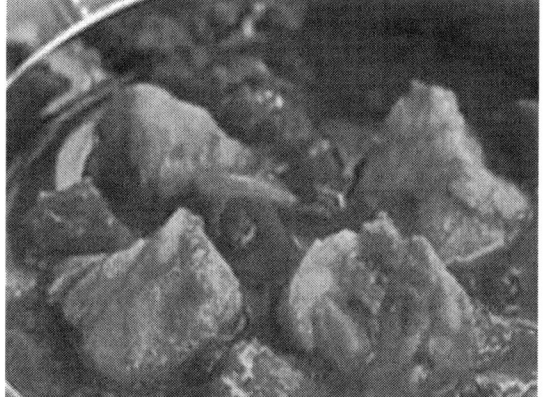

- 1 tablespoon curry paste
- 1 teaspoon curry
- 1 cup cream
- 1-pound salmon fillet
- ¼ cup garlic clove
- ½ tablespoon salt
- 1 teaspoon cilantro
- ¼ cup of fish sauce
- ½ cup of water
- 1 onion
- 1 teaspoon red Chile flake
- 1 tablespoon fresh ginger

Directions

1. Chop the salmon fillet roughly and transfer it to the pressure cooker.
2. Combine the cream and fish sauce in a mixing bowl.
3. Sprinkle the liquid mixture with the curry paste and curry and blend until smooth. Peel the garlic cloves and onion.
4. Chop the vegetables and add them to the cream mixture.
5. Grate the ginger and add the ginger, chili flakes, water, salt, and cilantro and mix well. Pour it onto the chopped salmon and coat the fish well.
6. Add the curried fish to the pressure cooker.
7. Close the lid and set the pressure cooker mode to "Pressure. Cook the dish for 10 minutes.
8. When the cooking time ends, release the remaining pressure and open the lid. Transfer the dish to serving bowls.

Nutritional Information: Calories: 264, Fat: 16.2g, Carbohydrates: 7.9g, Protein: 22g

Calamari in Tomato Sauce

Servings: 4

Prep time: 23 minutes

Ingredients:

- 12 ounces calamari
- 1 white onion
- 1 teaspoon cilantro
- 3 garlic cloves
- 1 teaspoon ground ginger
- ¼ cup fish stock
- 1 teaspoon fresh thyme
- ¼ cup wine
- ¼ cup of water
- 1 tablespoon olive oil
- 3 medium tomatoes
- ½ teaspoon ground white pepper
- 1 teaspoon lime juice

Directions:

1. Wash the calamari carefully and peel it.
2. Slice the calamari into medium-thick slices. Slice the garlic cloves, dice the onion, and c. hop the fresh thyme and tomatoes.
3. Set the pressure cooker to "Sauté" mode. Put the sliced calamari into the pressure cooker and sprinkle it with the olive oil. Sauté the dish for 5 minutes.
4. Add the garlic, onion, thyme, and tomatoes to the pressure cooker. Sprinkle the dish with the water, wine, ground ginger, lime juice, and fish stock, stir well, and close the lid.

5. Set the pressure cooker to "Sauté" mode. Stew the dish for 8 minutes. Remove the cooked calamari from the pressure cooker. Serve the dish hot.

Nutritional Information: calories 238, fat 6.1g, carbs 16.64g, protein 29g

Tomato and Shrimp Medley

Servings: 4

Preparation Time: 15 minutes

Ingredients

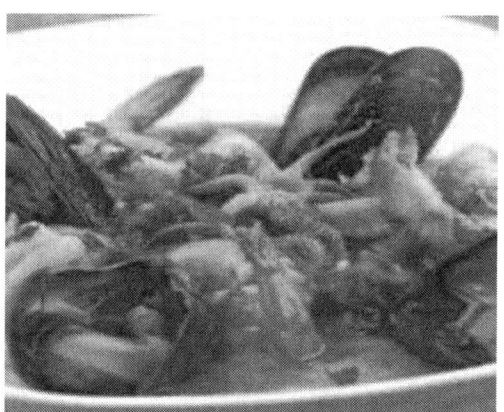

- 3 tablespoons unsalted butter
- 1 tablespoon garlic
- ½ teaspoon red pepper flakes
- 1 and ½ cup onion, chopped
- 1 can (14 and ½ ounces) tomatoes, diced
- 1 teaspoon dried oregano
- 1 teaspoon salt
- 1-pound frozen shrimp, peeled
- 1 cup crumbled feta cheese
- ½ cup black olives, sliced
- ½ cup parsley, chopped

Directions

1. Pre-heat your Ninja Foodi by setting in in the Sauté mode on HIGH settings, add butter and let it melt
2. Add garlic, pepper flakes, cook for 1 minute
3. Add onion, tomato, oregano, salt and stir well
4. Add frozen shrimp. Lock lid and cook on HIGH pressure for 1 minute
5. Quick release pressure
6. Mix shrimp with tomato broth, let it cool and serve with a sprinkle of feta, olives and parsley

Nutritional Information: Calories: 361, Fat: 22g, Carbohydrates: 11g, Protein: 30g

The Smoked White Fish

Servings: 4

Preparation Time: 2hrs 10 minutes

Ingredients

- 2 pounds Whitefish fillets, raw
- 1 tablespoon onion powder
- ½ teaspoon cumin
- 1 tablespoon paprika
- 1 tablespoon garlic powder
- 1 tablespoon olive oil
- Fresh lemon juice
- Fresh cilantro, chopped
- Salt and pepper to taste

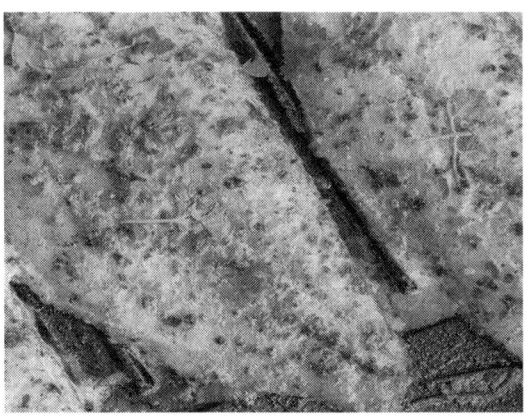

Directions

1. Set up your Ninja Foodi to 200 degrees F on a low heat setting
2. Use olive oil to brush the fish fillets
3. Add cumin, garlic powder, onion powder, paprika, salt, and pepper in a bowl and mix them well
4. Rub this prepared seasoning all over the pork from all the sides
5. Spray some olive oil more on the fillets
6. Put the seasoned fillets on the rack and put it inside the Ninja Foodi at a low temperature
7. Cook for 2 hours
8. Garnish it with chopped cilantro and fresh lemon juice
9. Serve and enjoy!

Nutritional Information: Calories: 142, Fat: 2g, Carbohydrates: 0g, Protein: 30g

Seafood Paella

Servings: 5

Prep time: 25 minutes

Ingredients:

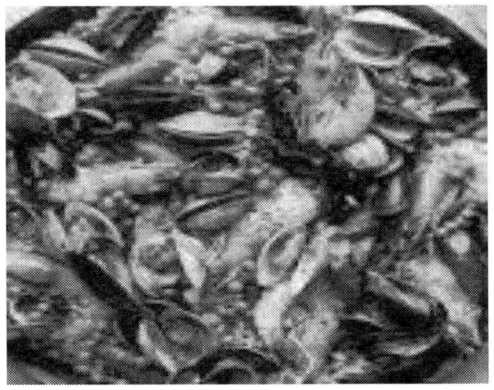

- 1 cup cauliflower rice
- 8 ounces shrimp
- 5 ounces mussels
- 2 cups fish stock
- 1 cup of water
- 1 tablespoon of sea salt
- 1 small chile pepper
- 1 teaspoon curry
- 1 teaspoon turmeric
- 1 tablespoon oregano
- 1 tablespoon fish sauce
- 1 teaspoon paprika
- 3 garlic cloves 1 tablespoon butter

Directions:

1. Peel the shrimp and combine them with the mussels. Place the seafood into the pressure cooker.
2. Add cauliflower rice, salt, curry, turmeric, oregano, and paprika and stir well.
3. Combine the fish stock, fish sauce, and butter together in a mixing bowl and blend well. Pour water mixture into the pressure cooker.
4. Peel the garlic and slice it. Chop the chile pepper. Sprinkle the cauliflower rice mixture with the sliced garlic and chopped chile pepper.
5. Stir briefly using a wooden spoon. Close the pressure cooker lid and set the pressure cooker mode to "Steam". Cook for 15 minutes.

6. When the dish is cooked, remove the food from the pressure cooker. Transfer the paella to a serving bowl.

Nutritional Information: calories 130, fat 4.7g, carbs 4.9, protein 16.8

Lemony Tuna Bites

Servings: 4

Preparation Time: 20 minutes

Ingredients

- 1-pound tuna; skinless, boneless and cubed
- 1/4 cup butter; melted
- 2 tablespoons fresh lemon juice
- 3 tablespoons cilantro; chopped.
- Salt and black pepper around the taste

Directions

1. Set the Foodi on Sauté mode add the butter, heat it down, add the tuna and sear it for 1 minute on either side.
2. Add other ingredients, position pressure lid on and cook on High for 8 minutes.
3. Release pressure naturally for 10 minutes, divide the tuna mix into bowls and serve.

Nutritional Information: Calories: 257, Fat: 10.74g, Carbohydrates: 2.76g, Protein: 36g

Cool Lemon and Dill Fish Packages

Servings: 4

Preparation Time: 25 minutes

Ingredients

- 2 tilapia cod fillets
- Salt, pepper and garlic powder to taste
- 2 sprigs fresh dill
- 4 slices lemon
- 2 tablespoons butter

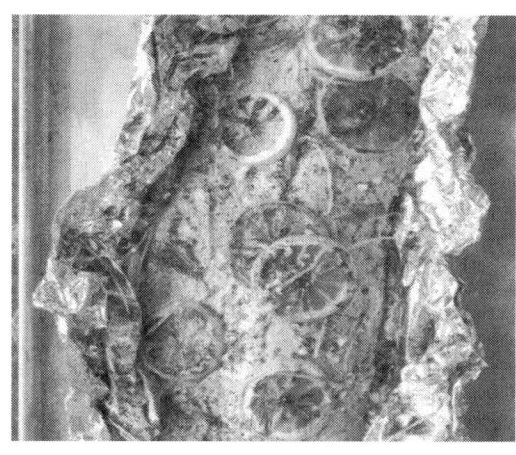

Directions

1. Lay out 2 large squares of parchment paper
2. Place fillet in center of each parchment square and season with salt, pepper and garlic powder
3. On each fillet, place 1 sprig of dill, 2 lemon slices, 1 tablespoon butter
4. Place trivet at the bottom of your Ninja Foodi
5. Add 1 cup water into the pot
6. Close parchment paper around fillets and fold to make a nice seal
7. Place both packets in your pot
8. Lock lid and cook on HIGH pressure for 5 minutes
9. Quick release pressure
10. Serve and enjoy!

Nutritional Information: Calories: 259, Fat: 11g, Carbohydrates: 8g, Protein: 20g

Fish Pie

Servings: 8

Prep time: 45 minutes

Ingredients:

- 1 tablespoon curry paste
- 1 teaspoon curry
- 1 cup cream
- 1 pound salmon fillet
- ¼ cup garlic clove
- ½ tablespoon salt
- 1 teaspoon cilantro
- 1 teaspoon olive oil
- ¼ cup of fish sauce
- 1 onion
- 1 teaspoon red chili flakes
- 1 tablespoon fresh ginger
- 10 ounces keto dough

Directions:

1. Roll the keto dough using a rolling pin. Spray the pressure cooker with the olive oil. Place the rolled dough into the pressure cooker.
2. Combine the curry paste, curry, cream, salt, cilantro, fish sauce, water, chili flakes, and fresh ginger in a mixing bowl and blend well and stir well.
3. Chop the salmon fillet and put it in the mixing bowl. Add curry paste mixture and mix well.
4. Put the fish mixture in the middle of the pie crust. Grate the fresh ginger and sprinkle the top of the pie.

5. Peel the onion, slice it, and add it to the top of the fish pie and close the lid. Set the pressure cooker to "Pressure" mode. Cook the dish on for 30 minutes.
6. When the pie is cooked, remove it from the pressure cooker and slice it. Serve the pie warm.

Nutritional Information: calories 256, fat 8.5g, carbs 13g, protein 32.8g

Cumin Mackerel Fillets

Servings: 4

Preparation Time: 22 minutes

Ingredients

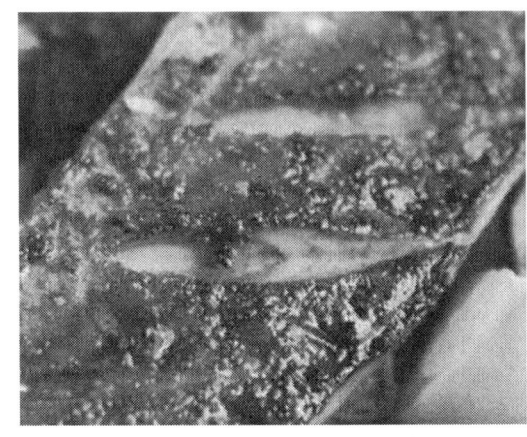

- 4 mackerel fillets; boneless
- 1 tablespoon canola oil
- 1 teaspoon garlic powder
- 1 teaspoon cumin; ground
- Juice of a single lime
- Salt and black pepper on the taste

Directions

1. In a bowl, mix the mackerel with all of those other ingredient and toss. Put the Foodi's basket in the device and add the fillets inside.
2. Cook the fish on Air Crisp mode at 370°F for 12 minutes, flipping the fillets halfway. Divide the fish between plates and serve with a side salad.

Nutritional Information: Calories: 233, Fat: 17g, Carbohydrates: 0g, Protein: 20g

Spicy Whitebait

Serves: 3

Prep time: 20 minutes

Ingredients:

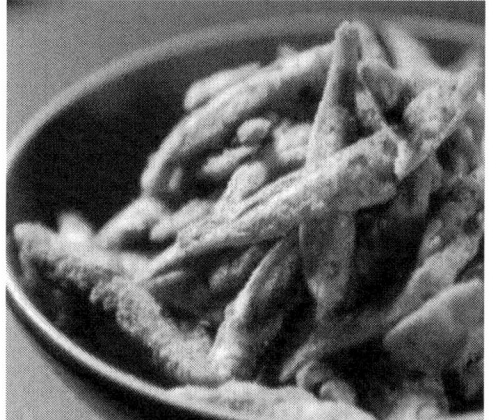

- 1 teaspoon red chile flakes
- 1 tablespoon sour cream
- 4 tablespoons garlic sauce
- 1 pound whitebait
- 3 tablespoons butter
- ½ teaspoon sage
- 1 teaspoon oregano
- 1 teaspoon olive oil
- ½ cup almond flour
- ¼ cup milk
- 1 egg
- ½ teaspoon ground ginger

Directions:

1. Make fillets from the whitebait. Combine the chile flakes, sage, oregano, and ground ginger in a bowl and mix well and stir.
2. Rub the whitebait fillets with the spice mixture. Let the fish rest for 5 minutes. Meanwhile, beat the egg in a separate bowl and whisk it.
3. Add the milk and flour and stir until smooth. Add the sour cream and stir. Dip the whitebait fillets in the egg mixture. Set the pressure cooker to "Pressure" mode.
4. Add the butter into the pressure cooker and melt it. Add the whitebait fillets and close the pressure cooker.

5. Cook the dish on for 10 minutes. When the cooking time ends, release the remaining pressure and open the pressure cooker lid. Transfer the whitebait in a serving plate.

Nutritional information: calories 472, fat 29.8g, carbs 7.4g, protein 43.2g

Heart-Throb Buttery Scallops

Servings: 4

Preparation Time: 25 minutes

Ingredients

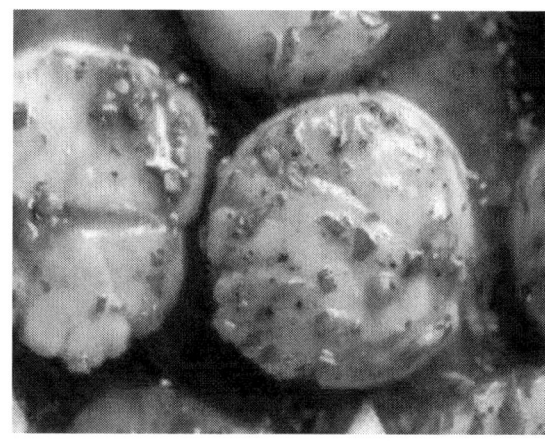

- 4 garlic cloves, minced
- 4 tablespoons fresh rosemary, chopped
- 2 pounds sea scallops
- ½ cup butter
- Salt and pepper to taste

Directions

1. Set your Ninja Foodi to Sauté mode and add butter and let it melt
2. Add rosemary, garlic and Sauté for 1 minute
3. Add sea scallops, salt and pepper
4. Sauté for 2 minutes more
5. Lock Crisping Lid and cook on "Air Crisp" mode for 3 minutes at 350 degrees F
6. Once done, serve and enjoy!

Nutritional Information: Calories: 279, Fat: 16g, Carbohydrates: 4g, Protein: 25g

Shrimp and Peas

Servings: 4

Preparation Time: 25 minutes

Ingredients

- 1-pound shrimp; peeled and deveined
- 5 ounces peas
- 1½ cups chicken stock
- 1 teaspoon essential olive oil
- 1 teaspoon sweet paprika
- Salt and black pepper for the taste

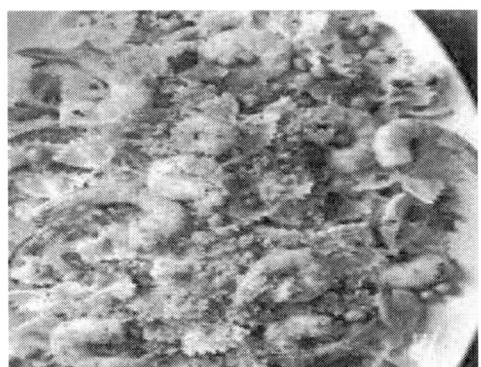

Directions

1. In your Foodi, mix every one of the ingredients, place the stress lid on and cook on High for 25 approximately minutes.
2. Release pressure to succeed naturally for 5 minutes, divide between plates and serve.

Nutritional Information: Calories: 165, Fat: 17g, Carbohydrates: 7g, Protein: 0g

Coconut Fish Curry

Servings: 4

Preparation Time: 25 minutes

Ingredients

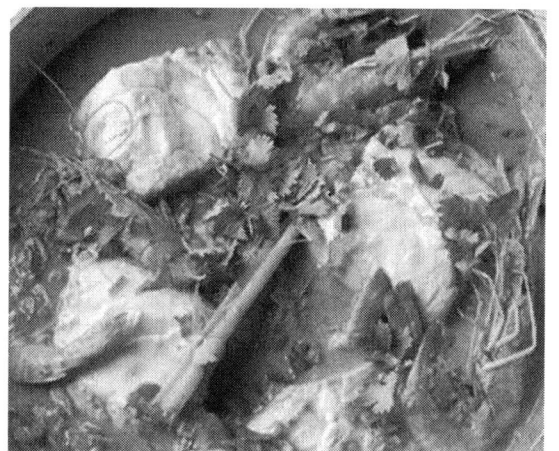

- 1 and ½ pounds white fish fillets, rinsed and cut into bite sized pieces
- 1 heaping cup cherry tomatoes
- 2 green chilies, sliced into strips
- 2 garlic cloves, finely chopped
- 1 tablespoon ginger, freshly grated
- 6 curry leaves such as bay leaves
- 1 tablespoon ground coriander
- 1 tablespoon ground cumin
- ½ teaspoon ground turmeric
- 1 teaspoon chili powder
- ½ teaspoon ground fenugreek
- 2 cups coconut milk, unsweetened
- 1 teaspoon olive oil
- Salt to taste
- Lemon juice to taste

Directions

1. Set your Ninja Foodi to Sauté mode and add oil and curry leaves
2. Gently fry for 1 minute, add onion, garlic, ginger and Sauté until onion are tender
3. Add coriander, turmeric, chili powder, fenugreek (all ground) and Sauté with onions for 1 minute

4. Deglaze pot with coconut milk, scraping browned bits
5. Add green chilies, tomatoes and fish and stir to coat
6. Lock lid and cook on HIGH pressure for 3 minutes, quick release pressure
7. Open lid and season with salt and lemon juice
8. Enjoy!

Nutritional information: Calories: 276, Fat: 21g, Carbohydrates: 4g, Protein: 18g

Monkfish Stew

Servings: 7

Prep time: 40 minutes

Ingredients:

- 1 pound monkfish fillet
- ½ cup white wine
- 1 teaspoon salt
- 1 teaspoon white pepper
- 1 medium carrot
- 2 white onions
- 1 cup fish stock
- 3 tablespoons fish sauce
- 1 tablespoon olive oil
- 1 teaspoon oregano
- ½ teaspoon fresh rosemary
- 1 cup of water
- 1 teaspoon sugar
- 1 teaspoon thyme
- 1 teaspoon coriander

Directions:

1. Chop the monkfish fillet roughly and sprinkle it with the salt, white pepper, fish sauce, oregano, fresh oregano, sugar, thyme, and coriander and stir well.
2. Let the fish rest for 5 minutes. Peel the onions and carrot and chop the vegetables. Set the pressure cooker to "Sauté" mode.
3. Put the chopped vegetables and monkfish into the pressure cooker. Sprinkle the mixture with the white wine, water, and olive oil.
4. Mix well and close the pressure cooker lid. Cook the dish on for 30 minutes.

5. When the stew is cooked, open the pressure cooker lid and let the stew rest for 10 minutes.
6. Transfer the stew to a serving bowl and serve.

Nutritional Information: calories 251, fat 14g, carbs 15g, protein 17g

Warm Cajun Bass Stew

Servings: 6

Preparation Time: 40 minutes

Ingredients

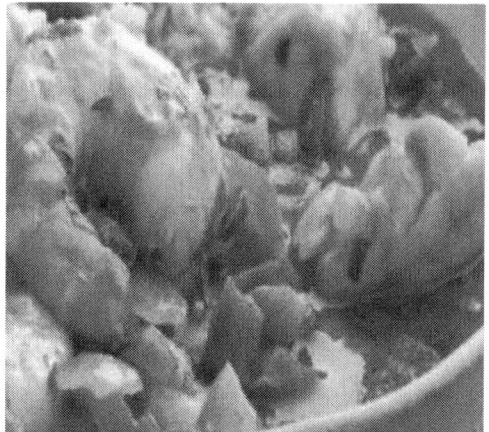

- 1-pound sea bass fillets, patted dry and cut into 2-inch chunks
- 3 tablespoons Cajun seasoning, divided
- ½ teaspoon salt
- 2 tablespoons extra virgin olive oil
- 2 yellow onion, diced
- 2 bell peppers, diced
- 4 celery stalks, diced
- 1 can (28 ounces) diced tomatoes, drained
- ¼ cup tomato paste
- 1 and ½ cups veggie broth
- 2 pounds large shrimp, peeled and deveined

Directions

1. Set your Pot to Sauté mode at a temperature of Medium-HIGH heat, let it pre-heat for 5 minutes
2. Season sea bass on both sides with 1 and ½ tablespoons Cajun seasoning and ¼ teaspoon salt
3. Put 1 tablespoon oil and sea bass in your pre-heated pot. Sauté for 4 minutes
4. Add remaining 1 tablespoon oil and onions to the pot and cook for 3 minutes, add bell peppers, celery, and 1 and ½ tablespoons Cajun seasoning to the pot. Cook for 2 minutes more

5. Add sea bass, diced tomatoes, tomato paste, broth to the pot, place the lid and seal the valves
6. Cook on HIGH pressure for 5 minutes, quick release the pressure once did
7. Set your pot to Sauté mode again with the temperature set at Medium-HIGH mode and add shrimp
8. Place lid and seal the pressure valve, cook for 4 minutes until the shrimp is opaque
9. Season with ¼ teaspoon salt and serve, enjoy!

Nutritional Information: Calories: 326, Fat: 10g, Carbohydrates: 9g, Protein: 46g

Cilantro Cod

Servings: 4

Preparation Time: 17 minutes

Ingredients

- 4 black cod fillets; boneless
- 2 garlic cloves; minced
- 4 tablespoons veggie stock
- 2 tablespoons cilantro; chopped.
- 1/2 teaspoon sweet paprika
- Salt and pepper for the taste

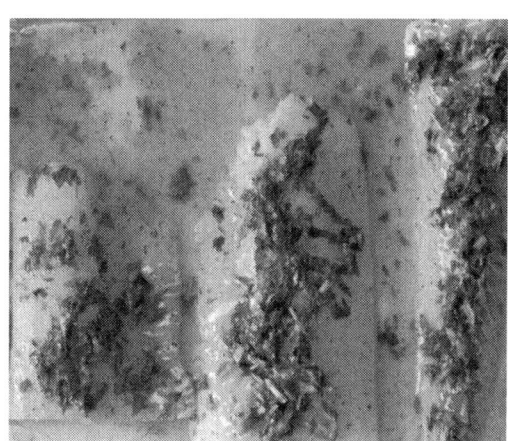

Directions

1. In your Foodi, mix each of the ingredients, place the pressure lid on and cook on High for 12 minutes.
2. Release pressure to ensure success fast for 5 minutes, divide the amalgamation between plates and serve.

The Great Lobster Bisque

Servings: 4

Preparation Time: 20 minutes

Ingredients

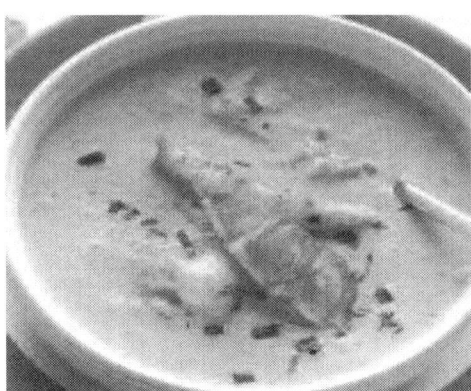

- 2 teaspoons unsalted butter
- 1 onion, chopped
- 1 tablespoon garlic, minced
- 1 tablespoon fresh ginger, minced
- 2 cups vegetable broth
- 1 cup tomatoes, chopped
- 3 cups cauliflower, chopped
- 2 tablespoons Keto-Friendly pesto
- ½ teaspoon salt
- 1 -2 teaspoons fresh ground black pepper
- 1-pound cooked lobster meat
- 1 cup heavy whip cream

Directions

1. Pre-heat your Ninja Foodi by setting to Sauté mode on HIGH settings
2. Once the inner pot is hot, add butter and let it heat up
3. Once the butter is shimmering, add onion, garlic and ginger. Sauté for 2-3 minutes
4. Add broth, stir, making sure to scrape the bottom of the pan to remove any browned bits
5. Add tomatoes, cauliflower, pesto, salt and pepper
6. Lock lid and cook on HIGH pressure for 4 minutes
7. Release pressure naturally over 10 minutes
8. Use an immersion blender to puree the veggies in the soup

9. Turn Sauté mode on and let the meat cook for a while, stir in cream and serve

Nutritional Information: Calories: 441, Fat: 30g, Carbohydrates: 10g, Protein: 30g

Sriracha Shrimp

Serves: 8

Prep time: 18 minutes

Ingredients:

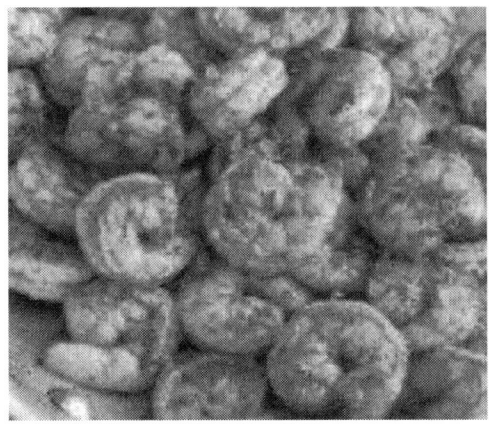

- 1 pound shrimp
- 3 tablespoons minced garlic
- 1 tablespoon sriracha
- 1 tablespoon sesame oil
- 1 teaspoon salt
- 1 teaspoon ground black pepper
- 1 teaspoon ground ginger
- ⅓ cup fish stock
- 1 tablespoon butter

Directions:

1. Peel the shrimp and combine them with the sriracha in a mixing bowl and stir well and sprinkle it with the sesame oil, minced garlic, salt, ground black pepper, ground ginger, and fish stock and stir well.
2. Toss everything well. Place the sriracha shrimp into the pressure cooker. Set the pressure cooker to "Pressure" mode.
3. Add the butter and close the pressure cooker lid. Cook the dish on for 8 minutes. When the dish is cooked, remove the food from the pressure cooker. Let the dish rest.
4. Let the dish rest briefly and serve.

Nutritional Information: calories 125, fat 5.4g, carbs 2.33g, protein 16g

Elegant Fish Curry

Servings: 4

Preparation Time: 10 minutes

Ingredients

- 2 tablespoons coconut oil
- 1 and ½ tablespoons fresh ginger, grated
- 2 teaspoons garlic, minced
- 1 tablespoon curry powder
- ½ teaspoon ground cumin
- 2 cups coconut milk
- 16 ounces firm white fish, cut into 1-inch chunks
- 1 cup kale, shredded
- 2 tablespoons cilantro, chopped

Directions

1. Pre-heat your Ninja Foodi to by selecting the Sauté mode and setting the temperature to HIGH heat
2. Add coconut oil and let it heat up, add ginger and garlic and Sauté for 2 minutes until light browned
3. Stir in curry powder, cumin, Sauté for 2 minutes until fragrant
4. Stir in coconut milk, reduce heat to low and simmer for 5 minutes
5. Lock lid and cook on LOW pressure for 4 minutes
6. Release pressure naturally over 10 minutes
7. Stir in kale and cilantro, simmer in Sauté mode for 2 minutes
8. Serve and enjoy!

Nutritional Information: Calories: 416, Fat: 31g, Carbohydrates: 5g, Protein: 26g

Almond Cod Fillets

Servings: 4

Preparation Time: 25 minutes

Ingredients

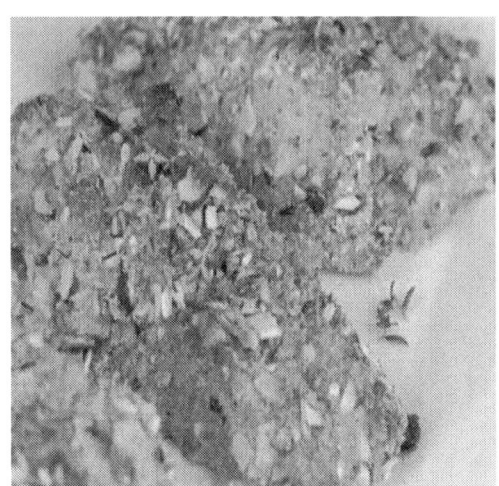

- 1 pound frozen cod fish fillets
- 2 garlic cloves, halved
- 1 cup chicken broth
- ½ cup packed parsley
- 2 tablespoons oregano
- 2 tablespoons almonds, sliced
- ½ teaspoon paprika

Directions

1. Take the fish out of freezer and let it defrost
2. Take a food processor and stir in garlic, oregano, parsley, paprika, 1 tablespoon almond and process
3. Set your Ninja Foodi to "SAUTE" mode and add olive oil, let it heat up
4. Add remaining almonds and toast, transfer to a towel
5. Pour broth in pot and add herb mixture
6. Cut fish into 4 pieces and place in a steamer basket, transfer steamer basket to the pot
7. Lock lid and cook on HIGH pressure for 3 minutes
8. Quick release pressure once done
9. Serve steamer fish by pouring over the sauce

Nutritional Information: Calories: 246, Fat: 10g, Carbohydrates: 8g, Protein: 15g

Tuna and Shirataki Noodles Salad

Serves:

Preparation time: 22 minutes

Ingredients:

- 5 ounces Shirataki noodles
- 1 pound tuna
- 1 tablespoon olive oil
- 1 teaspoon ground black pepper
- 3 tablespoons sour cream
- 1 teaspoon ground ginger
- 5 tablespoon fish stock
- 1 tablespoon soy sauce
- 6 ounces Parmesan cheese
- 1 cup black olives
- 1 cup hot water

Directions:

1. Combine the ground black pepper and ground ginger together in a bowl and mix well and stir.
2. Chop the tuna and add it to the ground black pepper mixture, stirring well. Cut the cheese into the cubes. Set the pressure cooker to "Steam" mode.
3. Place the chopped tuna into the pressure cooker and cook it for 12 minutes. Combine the sliced black olives, cheese cubes, olive oil in the mixing bowl. Add soy sauce and fish stock. Sprinkle the mixture with the sour cream.
4. When the tuna is cooked, release the pressure and open the instant lid. Chill the chopped tuna. Combine hot water and noodles together and let them sit for 15 minutes.
5. Rinse the noodles and place them in the black olive mixture.

6. Add the chilled chopped tuna and toss the salad gently. Transfer the salad to serving bowls.

Nutritional Information: calories 301, fat 18.3g, carbs 3.3g, protein 30.2g

Cod with Broccoli, Lemon and Dill Mismash

Servings: 4

Preparation Time: 20 minutes

Ingredients

- 1 pound, 1-inch thick frozen cod fillets
- 2 cups broccoli
- 1 cup water
- Dill weed
- Lemon pepper to taste
- Dash of salt

Directions

1. Cut fish into four pieces
2. Season fish pieces with lemon pepper, salt, dill weed
3. Add 1 cup water to the Ninja Foodi
4. Lower down steamer basket and add fish, broccoli florets to the steamer basket
5. Lock lid and cook on LOW pressure for 2 minutes
6. Quick release pressure
7. Serve!

Nutritional Information: Calories: 463, Fat: 33g, Carbohydrates: 12g, Protein: 25g

Cod and Celery Stew

Servings: 4

Preparation Time: 30 minutes

Ingredients

- 4 cod fillets; skinless, boneless and cubed
- 1 yellow onion; chopped.
- 1 cup celery; chopped.
- 1 tablespoon butter; melted
- 1 teaspoon sweet paprika
- Salt and black pepper around the taste

Directions

1. Set the Foodi on Sauté mode, add the butter, heat it, add the onion and celery, stir and cook for 5 minutes.
2. Add other ingredients, position the pressure lid on and cook on High for quarter-hour. Release the load naturally for ten mins, divide the stew into bowls and serve.

Nutritional Information: Calories: 417, Fat: 20g, Carbohydrates: 17g, Protein: 39g

Crunchy Cod

Serves: 4

Preparation time: 20 minutes

Ingredients:

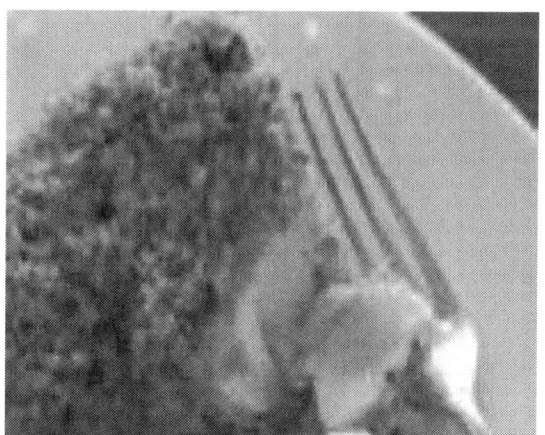

- 12 ounces cod fillet
- 3 eggs
- 1 cup coconut flour
- ⅓ cup pork rinds
- 1 teaspoon salt
- 2 tablespoons olive oil
- 1 teaspoon ground white pepper
- 1 teaspoon ground ginger
- 1 tablespoon turmeric
- 2 teaspoons sesame seeds
- ¼ teaspoon red chili flakes

Directions:

1. Whisk the eggs in a mixing bowl using a hand mixer. Add the coconut flour and continue to mix the mixture until smooth.
2. Sprinkle the cod fillets with the salt, ground ginger, ground white pepper, and chili flakes. Add turmeric and mix well. Dip the cod fillets in the egg mixture. Sprinkle the fish with the pork rinds and sesame seeds.
3. Pour olive oil into the pressure cooker and preheat it on the "Sauté" mode. Add the cod fillets and cook them for 5 minutes on each side.
4. When the cod fillets are cooked, remove them from the pressure cooker and transfer the dish to paper towel drain. Rest briefly before serving.

Nutritional Information: calories 198, fat 12g, carbs 3.5g, protein 19.9g

Butter Dredged "Rich" Lobster

Servings: 4

Preparation Time: 35 minutes

Ingredients

- 6 Lobster Tails
- 4 garlic cloves
- ¼ cup butter

Directions

1. Preheat the Ninja Foodi to 400 degrees F at first
2. Open the lobster tails gently by using kitchen scissors
3. Remove the lobster meat gently from the shells but keep it inside the shells
4. Take a plate and place it
5. Add some butter in a pan and allow it melt
6. Put some garlic cloves in it and heat it over medium-low heat
7. Pour the garlic butter mixture all over the lobster tail meat
8. Let the fryer to broil the lobster at 130 degrees F
9. Remove the lobster meat from Ninja Foodi and set aside
10. Use a fork to pull out the lobster meat from the shells entirely
11. Pour some garlic butter over it if needed
12. Serve!

Nutritional Information: Calories: 160, Fat: 3g, Carbohydrates: 1g, Protein: 20g

Shrimp and Tomatoes

Servings: 2

Preparation Time: 15 minutes

Ingredients

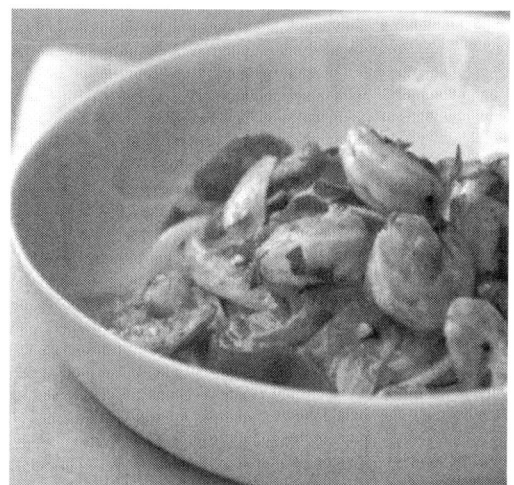

- 1-pound shrimp; peeled and deveined
- 1 cup canned tomatoes; chopped.
- 1 tablespoon essential extra virgin olive oil
- Salt and black pepper towards taste

Directions

1. Put the reversible rack inside Foodi, add the baking pan inside, add every one of the ingredients inside, set the product on Baking mode and cook at 380°F for 10 minutes.
2. Divide into bowls and serve.

Nutritional Information: Calories: 406.2, Fat: 10.7g, Carbohydrates: 3.8g, Protein: 2.8g

Spicy Flounder

Servings: 2

Preparation Time: 20 minutes

Ingredients

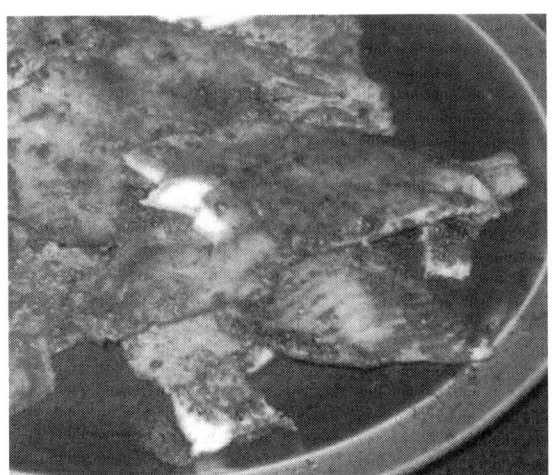

- 1 tbsp paprika
- 2 tsp salt
- 1 tsp ground black pepper
- 1 tsp chili powder
- 1 tsp onion powder
- 1 tsp garlic powder
- 1 tsp ground cumin
- 2 filets Flounder, about 1 pound
- 1 tbsp olive oil

Directions

1. Mix all of the spices together in a bowl and set aside
2. Rub the flounder with olive oil and then coat in the spice seasoning
3. Place the spiced flounder in the cook and crisp basket and turn the Ninja Foodi to 375 degrees. Place the basket in the Foodi and set the timer for 15 minutes.
4. Serve while hot straight out of the pot

Nutritional Information: Calories: 351, Fat: 12g, Carbohydrates: 6g, Protein: 51g

Lemon Pepper Salmon

Servings: 2

Preparation Time: 15 minutes

Ingredients

- 2 tbsp butter
- 1/3 cup lemon juice
- ½ cup water
- 1-pound Salmon, de boned
- ½ ground black pepper

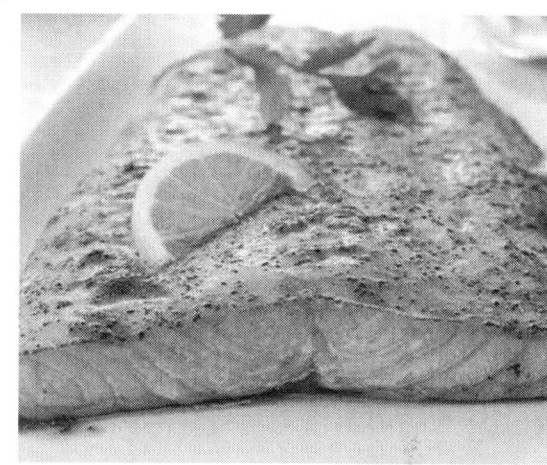

Directions

1. Add all the ingredients into the cook and crisp basket and place the basket inside the Ninja Foodi
2. Place the pressure cooker lid on top of the pot and close the pressure valve to the seal position. Set the pressure cooker function to higher heat and set the timer for 3 minutes
3. Once the cooking cycle is complete, release the pressure quickly by carefully opening the steamer valve. Enjoy while hot.

Nutritional Information: Calories: 314, Fat: 14g, Carbohydrates: 8g, Protein: 42g

Chapter Nine: Keto Ninja Foodi Pork and Beef Recipes

Beef Jerky

Servings: 6

Preparation Time: 15 minutes

Ingredients

- ½ pound beef, sliced into 1/8" thick strips
- ½ cup soy sauce
- 2 tbsp Worcestershire sauce
- 2 tsp ground black pepper
- 1 tsp onion powder
- ½ tsp garlic powder
- 1 tsp kosher salt

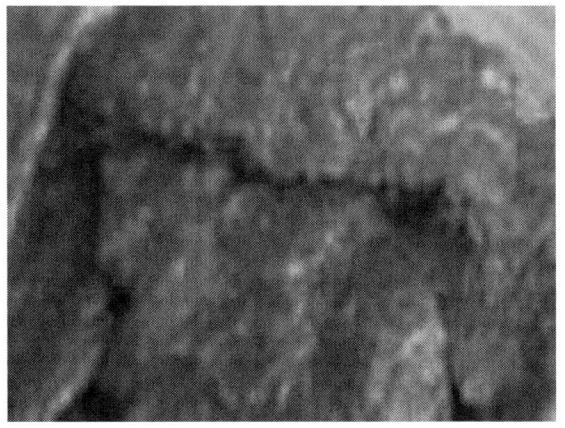

Directions

1. Place all the ingredients in a large Ziploc bag and seal shut. Shake to mix, then leave in the fridge overnight
2. Lay the strips on the dehydrator trays, being careful not to overlap them
3. Place the cook and crisp lid on and set the temperature for 135 degrees for 7 hours. Once done, store in an airtight container

Nutritional Information: Calories: 62, Fat: 7g, Carbohydrates: 2g, Protein: 9g

Baked Thyme Pork Stew

Servings: 4

Preparation Time: 40 minutes

Ingredients

- 1-pound pork stew meat, cubed
- 1 cup beef stock
- 2 garlic cloves, minced
- 2 teaspoons thyme, chopped.
- 2 tablespoons extra virgin essential olive oil
- Salt and black pepper towards taste

Directions

1. Put the reversible rack inside Foodi, add the baking pan inside and mix all the ingredients inside pan.
2. Cook on Baking mode at 390°F for thirty minutes.
3. Divide the stew into bowls and serve.

Nutritional Information: Calories: 198, Fat: 11.2g, Carbohydrates: 0,6g, Protein: 21.8g

Pork and Adobo Sauce

Servings: 4

Preparation Time: 35 minutes

Ingredients

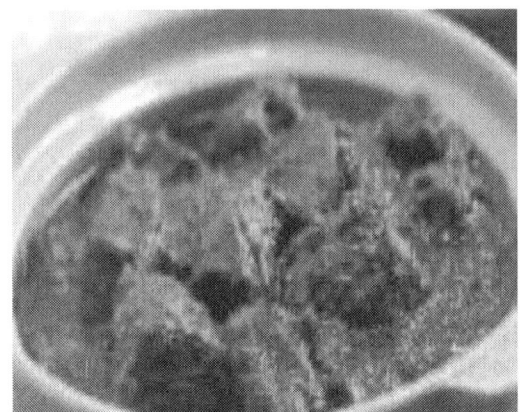

- 1-pound pork stew meat, cubed
- 1/2 cup tomato sauce
- 2 garlic cloves, minced
- 2 tablespoons extra virgin olive oil
- 1 teaspoon ginger, grated
- 2 teaspoons adobo sauce
- Salt and black pepper for the taste

Directions

1. Set the Foodi on Sauté mode, add the oil, heat, add the ginger, garlic combined with the meat and sauté for 5 minutes.
2. Add other ingredients, position the stress lid on and cook on High for 20 minutes.
3. Release the load naturally for ten mins, divide into bowls and serve.

Nutritional Information: Calories: 165, Fat: 9.4g, Carbohydrates: 3.43g, Protein: 14.93g

Beef Stew

Servings: 4

Preparation Time: 12 minutes

Ingredients

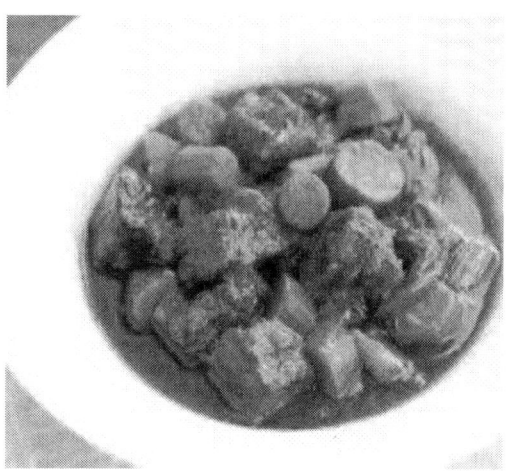

- 1-pound Beef Roast
- 4 cups beef broth
- 3 cloves of garlic, chopped
- 1 carrot, chopped
- 2 celery stalks, chopped
- 2 tomatoes, chopped
- ½ white onion, chopped
- ¼ tsp salt
- 1/8 tsp ground black pepper

Directions

1. Add all the ingredients to the pot and place pressure cooker lid on the Ninja Foodi
2. Cook on high pressure for 10 minutes. Do a quick steam release and remove the lid
3. Shred the beef using 2 forks
4. Serve while hot or freeze to use another day

Nutritional Information: Calories: 211, Fat: 7g, Carbohydrates: 2g, Protein: 10g

Beef Ragout

Servings: 10

Prep time: 50 minutes

Ingredients

- 2 pounds beef brisket
- 2 carrots
- 4 white onion
- 1 teaspoon sugar
- 3 cups of water
- 1 cup cherry tomatoes
- 1 tablespoon fresh thyme
- ¼ cup fresh dill
- ½ cup fresh parsley
- 1 cup cream
- 1 cup tomato juice
- 5 ounces fennel
- 11 teaspoon fresh rosemary
- 1 tablespoon butter

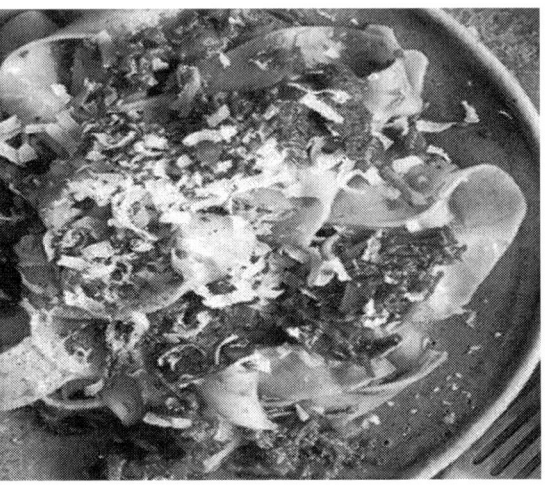

Directions:

1. Wash the thyme, dill, and parsley and chop them. Chop the beef brisket roughly. Wash the cherry tomatoes and cut them into halves. Chop the fennel.
2. Peel the onions and carrots and chop them roughly.
3. Place all the ingredients into the pressure cooker. Set the pressure cooker to «Sauté» mode. Add water, sugar, cream, tomato juice, fresh rosemary, and butter to the pressure cooker and stir well.

4. Close the pressure cooker lid and cook the beef ragout for 35 minutes. When the dish is cooked, remove the food from the pressure cooker, let it rest briefly and serve.

Nutrition: calories 271, fat 19.5g, carbs 8.96g, protein 15g

Pork Chops and Basil Pesto

Servings: 4

Preparation Time: 35 minutes

Ingredients

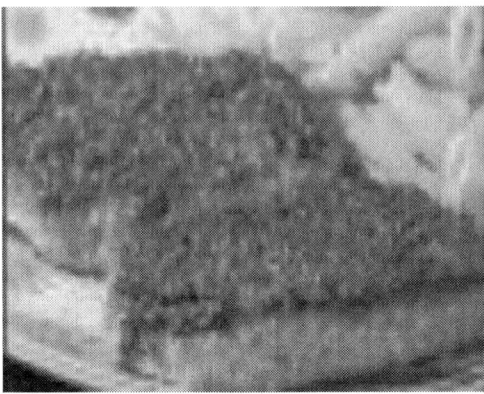

- 4 pork chops
- 1 tablespoon organic olive oil
- 3 tablespoons basil pesto
- Salt and black pepper for your taste

Directions

1. In a bowl, mix every one of the ingredients and toss. Put the chops as part of your Foodi's basket and cook on Air Crisp at 380°F for 25 minutes.
2. Divide between plates and serve with a side salad.

Nutritional Information: Calories: 241, Fat: 12g, Carbohydrates: 1g, Protein: 30g

Beef Stifado

Servings: 9

Prep time: 65 minutes

Ingredients

- 2 pounds beef rump
- 2 tablespoons tomato paste
- 1 teaspoon salt
- 1 cup onion
- 3 tablespoons olive oil
- ½ cup red wine
- 2 ounces bay leaf
- 1 teaspoon black-eyed peas
- 1 tablespoon ground ginger
- 1 teaspoon thyme
- 1 tablespoon cayenne pepper
- 4 tablespoons lemon juice
- 1 teaspoon cilantro
- 1 teaspoon oregano
- 1 teaspoon minced garlic

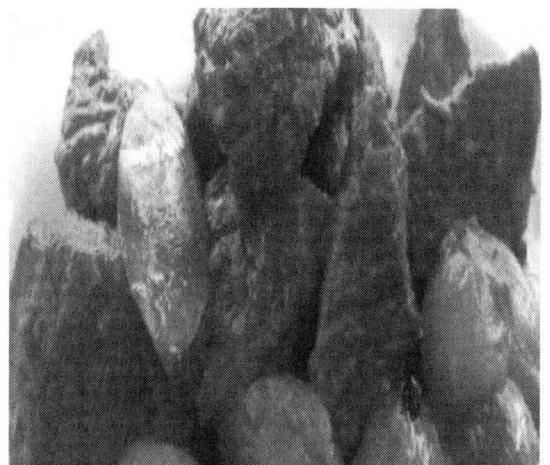

Directions:

1. Chop the beef rump and sprinkle it with salt. Peel the onions and slice them. Combine the sliced onions with the olive oil and stir well.
2. Combine the red wine, bay leaves, black-eyed peas, ground ginger thyme, cayenne pepper, lemon juice, cilantro, oregano, and minced garlic together in a mixing bowl.
3. Set the pressure cooker to "Sauté" mode. Add the sliced onion mixture to the pressure cooker and sauté for 10 minutes, stirring frequently.

4. Add the chopped beef rump and let it marinate for a few minutes. Stir well and close the pressure cooker lid. Cook the dish on "Sauté" mode for 40 minutes.
5. When the cooking time ends, open the pressure cooker lid and stir again. Transfer the dish to serving bowls.

Nutritional Information: calories 218, fat 11.3, fiber 2, carbs 8.07, protein 23

Beef Ribs

Servings: 4

Preparation Time: 50 minutes

Ingredients

- 2 pounds beef spare ribs, boneless
- 1 ½ cup beef broth
- ½ tsp ground black pepper
- 1 ½ tsp paprika
- 1 tsp onion powder
- 1 tsp garlic powder
- 1 cup tomato sauce
- 1 ½ tbsp butter, melted
- 2 tbsp apple cider vinegar
- 1 tbsp Worcestershire sauce
- 2 tbsp stevia powder
- ½ tsp onion powder
- ½ tsp salt

Directions

1. In a small bowl, mix together the melted butter, tomato sauce, vinegar, Worcestershire sauce, stevia, ½ tsp salt and ½ tsp onion powder
2. Place the ribs in Ninja Foodi bowl and sprinkle the remaining spices. Toss to coat completely.
3. Pour the home-made BBQ sauce into the bowl with the ribs and place the pressure cooker lid on top of the pot. Set the timer for 30 minutes at high heat. Once the cooking cycle is complete, let the pressure naturally release from the pot, about another 15 minutes.
4. Brush the ribs with the sauce from the bottom of the pot and then place the crisper lid on the pot. Set the temperature for 400 and set the timer for 10 minutes.

5. Let the ribs brown and then serve hot

Nutritional Information: Calories: 610, Fat: 46g, Carbohydrates: 6g, Protein: 41g

Lamb and Butternut Squash

Servings: 4

Preparation Time: 30 minutes

Ingredients

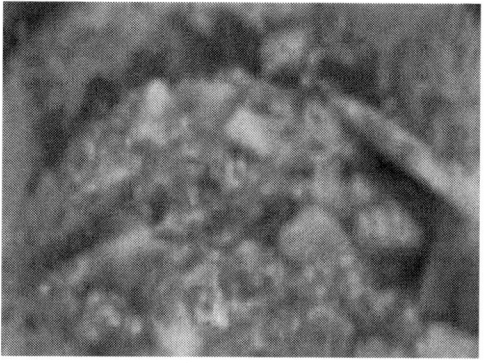

- 2 pounds lamb shoulder; cubed
- 1/2 cup beef stock
- 2 garlic cloves; minced
- 1 butternut squash; cut into wedges
- 2 red onions; chopped
- Juice of a single lemon
- 1 tablespoon essential olive oil
- 1 tablespoon cilantro; chopped.
- Salt and black pepper towards the taste

Directions

1. Put the reversible rack inside the Foodi, add the baking pan inside and mix every one of the ingredients inside.
2. Cook on Baking mode at 380°F for 25 minutes, divide everything between plates and serve.

Beef and Brussels Sprouts

Servings: 4

Preparation Time: 35 minutes

Ingredients

- 1-pound beef stew meat, cubed
- 1/2-pound Brussels sprout
- 1/4 cup beef stock
- 1 tablespoon sweet paprika
- 1 tablespoon essential olive oil
- Salt and black pepper for your taste

Directions

1. Set the Foodi on Sauté mode, add the oil, get hot, add the meat as well as the paprika and brown for 5 minutes.
2. Add the sprouts as well as the stock, squeeze pressure lid on and cook on High for 25 minutes. Release pressure to ensure success fast for 5 minutes, divide into bowls and serve.

NY Strip Steak

Servings: 2

Preparation Time: 10 minutes

Ingredients

- 24 ounces NY strip steak
- ½ tsp ground black pepper
- 1 tsp salt

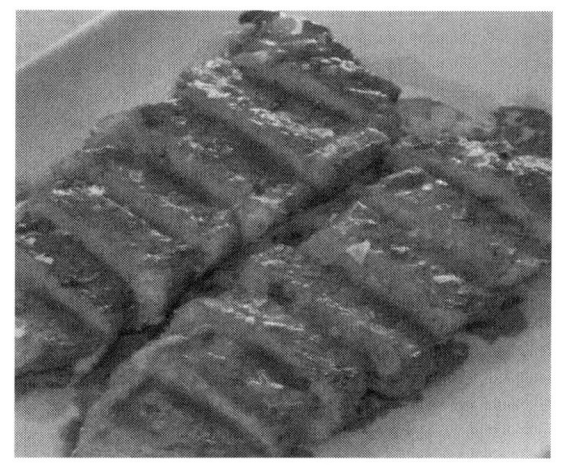

Directions

1. Place the steaks on the metal trivet in the Ninja Foodi and sprinkle the salt and pepper over the top
2. Add 1 cup of water to the pot, below the steaks
3. Put the pressure lid on the pot and set to cook at high pressure for 1 minute. Once the timer is done, release the pressure quickly by opening the steamer valve carefully
4. Place the air crisp lid on the pot and select the broil function and set the timer for 8 minutes for a medium cooked steak
5. Remove from pot and serve hot

Nutritional Information: Calories: 503, Fat: 46g, Carbohydrates: 1g, Protein: 46g

Beef Brisket with Red Wine

Servings: 6

Preparation time: 55 minutes

Ingredients

- 1 cup sweet red wine
- 1 lemon
- 1 teaspoon ground black pepper
- ½ teaspoon cinnamon
- 1 teaspoon ground ginger
- 1 teaspoon cilantro
- 1 tablespoon butter
- 1 pound beef brisket
- 1 cup of water
- 1 teaspoon turmeric

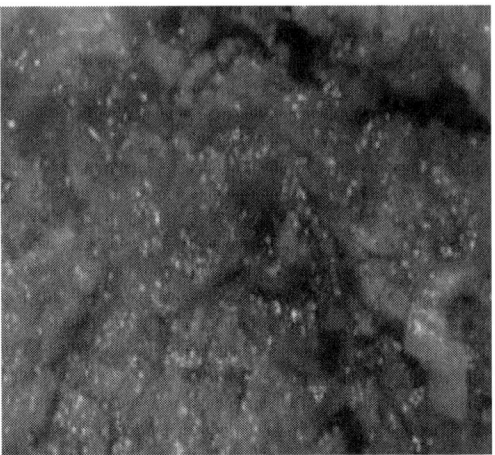

Directions:

1. Place the beef brisket in a mixing bowl. Combine the wine with the ground black pepper, cinnamon, ground ginger, cilantro, and turmeric in another bowl and stir well.
2. Set the pressure cooker to "Sauté" mode. Pour the wine mixture in the brisket bowl and let it sit for 15 minutes.
3. Transfer the brisket to the pressure cooker and add the water. Slice the lemon and add it to the meat mixture. Close the pressure cooker lid and cook for 40 minutes.
4. When the cooking time ends, open the pressure cooker and remove the meat from the wine mixture. Slice the cooked meat and serve.

Nutritional Information: calories 182, fat 13.3g, carbs 2.2g, protein 11g

Pork and Sweet Onion

Servings: 4

Preparation Time: 35 minutes

Ingredients

- 1½ pounds pork tenderloin, sliced
- 1/2 cup beef stock
- 1 tablespoon extra-virgin olive oil
- 3 sweet onions, chopped
- Salt and black pepper around the taste

Directions

1. Set the Foodi on Sauté mode, add the oil, get hot, add the onions and sauté for 5 minutes. Add the pork and the remaining ingredients, place the stress lid on and cook High for 25 minutes.
2. Release pressure to have success naturally for ten mins, divide everything between plates and serve.

Nutritional Information: Calories: 304.7, Fat: 15g, Carbohydrates: 12.5g, Protein: 28.5g

Short Ribs and Veggies

Servings: 2

Preparation Time: 16 minutes

Ingredients

- 3 pounds bone in beef short ribs
- 1 tsp ground black pepper
- 2 tsp salt
- 1 cup chopped onions
- ¼ cup Marsala
- ½ cup beef broth
- 2 Tbsp stevia
- 4 cloves garlic, chopped
- 1 tbsp chopped thyme
- 2 parsnips, chopped
- 1 cup pearl onions
- 1 cup chopped beets

Direction

1. Season ribs with the salt and pepper and then add to the Ninja Foodi pot with 1 tbsp of oil. Select the sear function and let the ribs sear for 5 minutes, flip and sear for 5 minutes.
2. Add the onion, wine, broth, stevia, garlic and thyme and place the pressure cooker lid on the Foodi. Set the pressure to high and the timer to 40 minutes. Once the timer is complete, quickly release the steam and open the lid.
3. Place the reversible rack over the top of the ribs in the pot. Place the veggies on the rack and drizzle with some extra oil
4. Close the crisper lid and set the temperature to 350 for 15 minutes

5. Remove the veggies and ribs and set aside. Press the sauté function and let the sauce in the pot cook for two more minutes before serving with the ribs and veggies

Nutritional Information: Calories: 506, Fat: 27g, Carbohydrates: 14g, Protein: 47g

Parmesan Beef Meatloaf

Servings: 6

Prep time: 30 minutes

Ingredients

- 8 ounces Parmesan cheese
- 3 eggs
- 1 pound ground beef
- 1 tablespoon tomato paste
- 1 teaspoon ground black pepper
- 1 tablespoon salt
- 4 tablespoons butter
- 1 tablespoon coconut flour
- 1 teaspoon cilantro
- 1 large onion
- 1 teaspoon minced garlic
- 2 tablespoons olive oil

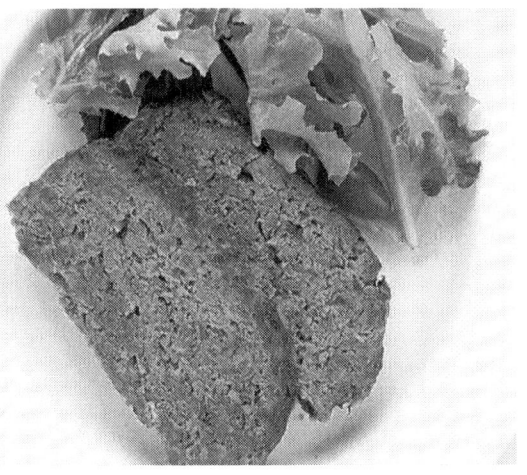

Directions:

1. Peel the onion and chop it roughly. Transfer the onion in the blender and puree until smooth. Combine the onion with the ground black pepper, salt, tomato paste, minced garlic, coconut flour, and cilantro and stir well.

2. Combine the spice mixture with the ground beef. Beat the eggs in a separate bowl. Combine the eggs and ground beef mixture together in a mixing bowl until fully combined. Form a loaf shape from the meat mixture and wrap it in aluminum foil. Set the pressure cooker to "Steam" mode.

3. Put the meatloaf in the trivet and place the trivet into the pressure cooker. Cook for 20 minutes. Grate the Parmesan cheese. When the cooking time ends, remove the meatloaf from the pressure cooker and discard it from aluminum foil. Sprinkle the meatloaf with the olive oil and grated cheese.
4. Transfer the dish to the pressure cooker and cook it on "Pressure" mode for 2 minutes. Remove the dish from the pressure cooker, cut into pieces, and serve.

Nutritional Information: calories 420, fat 27.6g, carbs 5.4, protein 38.6

Pork and Red Cabbage

Servings: 4

Preparation Time: 35 minutes

Ingredients

- 1-pound pork stew meat, cubed
- 1 red onion, chopped
- 1/2 cup sour cream
- 1 red cabbage head, shredded
- 2 tablespoons essential organic olive oil
- Salt and black pepper for the taste

Directions

1. Set the Foodi on Sauté mode, add the oil, heat it down, add the onion and also the meat and brown for 5 minutes.
2. Add other ingredients, place pressure to succeed lid on and cook on High for 20 roughly minutes.
3. Release pressure naturally for ten mins, divide the amalgamation into bowls and serve.

Nutritional Information: Calories: 234.6, Fat: 18.4g, Carbohydrates: 8g, Protein: 24g

Cauliflower Corned Beef Harsh

Serves:6

Preparation time: 35 minutes

Ingredients

- 6 eggs
- 4 cup riced cauliflower
- 1 pound corned beef, diced
- ¼ cup milk
- 1 onion, chopped
- 3 tbsp butter
- 2 cups chopped cooked ham
- ½ cup shredded cheese

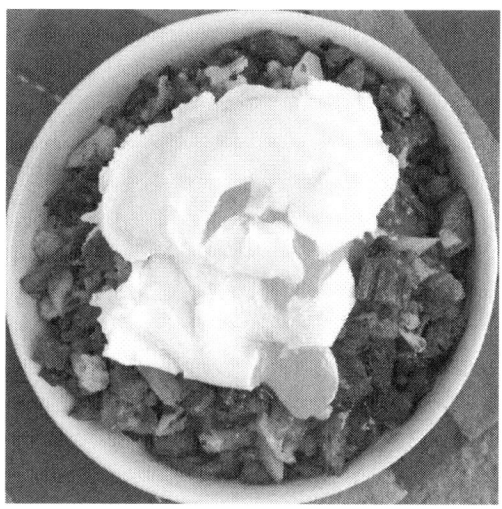

Directions

1. Press the sauté button on your Ninja Foodi and add butter and the onions. Cook stirring occasionally until the onions are soft, about 5 minutes
2. Add the riced cauliflower to the pot and stir. Turn on the air crisper for 15 minutes, turning the cauliflower halfway through
3. In a small bowl, mix the eggs and milk together then pour over the browned cauliflower.
4. Sprinkle the corned beef over the top of the egg mix
5. Press the air crisp button again and set the timer for 10 minutes
6. Sprinkle the cheddar cheese on top and close the lid of the Ninja Foodi for one minute to just melt the cheese. Serve while hot

Nutritional Information: Calories: 322, Fat: 26g, Carbohydrates: 3g, Protein: 20g

Ropa Vieja

Serves: 6

Preparation time: 35 minutes

Ingredients

- 2 pounds chuck roast
- 1 sliced onion
- 4 cloves garlic, minced
- 2 tsp oregano
- 1 tsp cumin
- 1 tsp paprika
- 2 tsp salt
- ½ tsp ground black pepper
- 1/8 tsp ground cloves
- 2 bay leaves
- 1 can diced tomatoes
- 2 red bels peppers

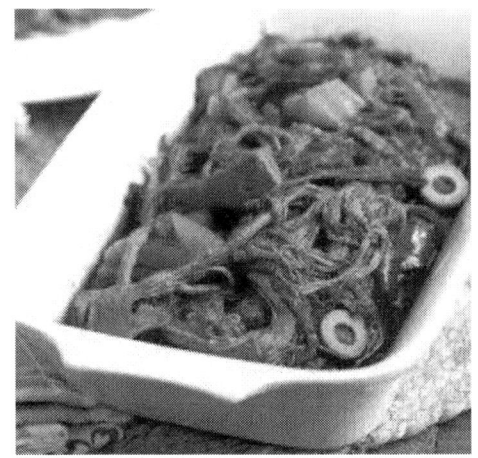

Directions

1. Add all the ingredients to the Ninja Foodi except the green bell peppers
2. Close the pressure cooker lid and seal the steamer valve. Set the timer for 90 minutes on low pressure
3. Allow the pressure to naturally release and then open the lid and shred the beef with two forks
4. Add the bell peppers and place the crisper lid on the pot. Cook at 350 for 5 minutes
5. Serve hot

Nutritional Information: Calories: 358, Fat: 26g, Carbohydrates: 3g, Protein: 28g

Lemon Pork Chops

Serves: 2

Preparation time: 15 minutes

Ingredients

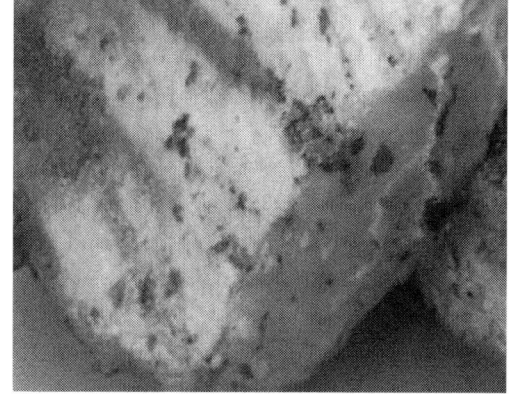

- ½ cup hot sauce
- ½ cup water
- 2 tbsp butter
- 1/3 cup lemon juice
- 1 pound pork cutlets
- ½ tsp paprika

Directions

1. Add all ingredients into the cook and crisp basket and place the basket inside the Ninja Foodi
2. Place the pressure cooker lid on top of the pot and close the pressure valve to the seal position.
3. Set the pressure cooker function to high heat and set the timer for 5 minutes
4. Once the cooking is complete, release pressure quickly by carefully opening the steamer valve. Enjoy while hot

Nutritional Information: Calories: 414, Fat: 21g, Carbohydrates: 3g, Protein: 50g

Sliced Beef with Saffron

Serves: 7

Prep time: 60 minutes

Ingredients

- 14 ounces beef brisket
- 1 tablespoon soy sauce
- 1 teaspoon oregano
- 1 teaspoon salt
- 3 ounces fresh saffron
- ½ teaspoon thyme
- 1 tablespoon ground coriander
- 1 cup chicken stock
- 1 tablespoon butter
- ⅓ teaspoon rosemary

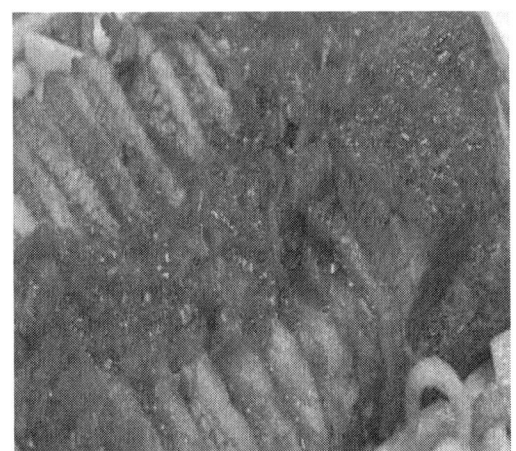

Directions:

1. Combine the oregano, salt, thyme, ground coriander, and rosemary together in a mixing bowl and stir well. Rub the beef brisket with the spice mixture and sprinkle the meat with soy sauce.
2. Chop the saffron, combine it with the butter and mix well. Set the pressure cooker to "Pressure" mode.
3. Add the saffron mixture to the pressure cooker and melt for 2 minutes. Add the brisket and chicken stock.
4. Close the pressure cooker lid and cook the dish on "Sauté" mode for 45 minutes.
5. When the cooking time ends, remove the meat from the pressure cooker and slice it before serving.

Nutritional Information: calories 184, fat 11.6g, carbs 9.93g, protein 11g

Pork with the Almonds and Sage

Servings: 11

Preparation time: 45 minutes

Ingredients

- 3 pounds pork loin
- 3 garlic cloves
- 3 carrots
- 3 tablespoons sage
- 5 tablespoon chicken stock
- 1 tablespoon olive oil
- 1 teaspoon lemon zest
- 1 tablespoon almond flakes
- 1 cup almond milk
- 1 tablespoons salt

Directions:

1. Rub the pork loin with the sage and leave it for 10 minutes. Peel the garlic cloves and carrots. Cut the carrots into halves.
2. Place the garlic cloves, carrots, and lemon zest into the pressure cooker. Add the olive oil, almond milk, salt, and almond flakes. Set the pressure cooker to "Sauté" mode. Place the pork into the pressure cooker.
3. Close the pressure cooker lid and cook the dish on meat mode for 40 minutes.
4. When the cooking time ends, open the pressure cooker lid, remove the cooked pork, and let it rest. Slice and serve warm.

Nutritional Information: calories 293, fat 15.4g, carbs 4.54g, protein 32g

Pork Schnitzel

Servings: 4

Preparation time: 25 minutes

Ingredients

- 1 pound boneless pork chops
- 1 cup pork rind
- 4 eggs
- 1 teaspoon salt
- 1 teaspoon ground black pepper
- 1 tablespoon olive oil
- 1 cup almond flour
- 1 tablespoon coconut milk

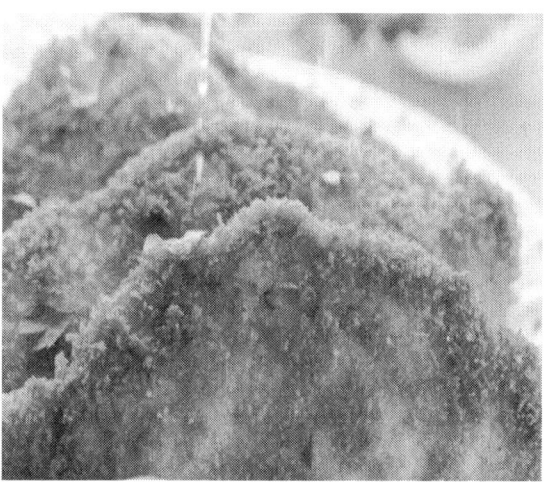

Directions:

1. Pound the pork chops flat using a meat mallet. Combine the salt and ground black pepper together in a mixing bowl and stir well.
2. Sprinkle the pork with the spice mixture. Beat the eggs, add coconut milk, and stir well. Set the pressure cooker to "Sauté" mode.
3. Pour the olive oil into the pressure cooker and preheat it. Dip the pork chops in the egg mixture, then dip the pork chops in the almond flour, and dip them in the egg mixture again. Finally, dip the pork chops into the pork rind and transfer the meat to the pressure cooker.
4. Sauté the pork chops for 5 minutes on each side. When the schnitzel is cooked, remove it from the pressure cooker and let it rest briefly before serving.

Nutritional Information: calories 745, fat 46.5g, carbs 5.9g, protein 69.1g

Crazy Greek Lamb Gyros

Serves: 8

Preparation time: 35 minutes

Ingredients

- 8 garlic cloves
- 1 and ½ teaspoon salt
- 2 teaspoons dried oregano
- 1 and ½ cups water
- 2 pounds lamb meat, ground
- 2 teaspoons rosemary
- ½ teaspoon pepper
- 1 small onion, chopped
- 2 teaspoons ground marjoram

Directions

1. Add onions, garlic, marjoram, rosemary, salt and pepper to a food processor
2. Process until combined well, add round lamb meat and process again
3. Press meat mixture gently into a loaf pan
4. Transfer the pan to your Ninja Foodi pot
5. Lock lid and select "Bake/Roast" mode
6. Bake for 25 minutes at 375 degrees F
7. Transfer to serving dish and enjoy!

Nutritional Information: Calories: 242, Fat: 15g, Carbohydrates: 2.4g, Protein: 21g

Conclusion

I thank you again for purchasing this book and I hope that you had as much fun reading it as I had writing it. I bid you farewell and encourage you to move forward with your amazing Keto journey with the shiny and revolutionary Ninja Foodi!

Printed in Great Britain
by Amazon